Heal Yourself and Your Loved Ones

Home Massage Therapy

Book 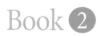 2

Heal Yourself and Your Loved Ones

Home Massage Therapy Book 2

Healing Society
6560 Highway 179, Ste.114
Sedona, AZ 86351
www.healingsociety.com
1–877–504–1106

Library Congress Control Number: 2004104232
ISBN-10: 1–932843–00–0
ISBN-13: 978–1–932843–00–2

Translated by Alexander Choi and Julie Han
Designed by Pishion
Printed in South Korea

If you are unable to order this book from your
local bookstores, you may order through
www.healingsociety.com or www.amazon.com.

Heal Yourself and Your Loved Ones

Home Massage Therapy
Book 2

DAHN HEALER SCHOOL

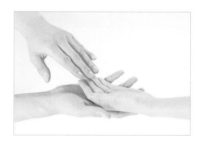

Healing Society

Preface

Many in this world are in search of magical medicines and renowned healers, but only few know the importance and benefits of the natural healing powers one has within oneself. Health is very closely within our reach. Dahnhak does not seek remedies from afar. It researches and develops programs to aid all individuals to easily discover natural self-healing mechanisms from within. Dahnhak Meridian Exercise, Dahn-Jon Breathing, Dahn-Diet, and meditation are all methods of improving circulation of 'Ki-energy' in our bodies, and to enhance our self-healing power.

Dahnhak Hwal-Gong is a healing method that does not require special training or skills. Anybody can utilize these life-supporting principles on a daily basis. By simply laying your bare hands on someone to heal you can open the hearts and minds of your family, neighbors and friends, and come to know the pure joy in giving and receiving love. Perhaps, today, we rely too much on synthesized medicine. We deprive ourselves of knowing the power of touch that transmits our loving warmth and devotion.

If you are suffering from being misunderstood by your friends and family, we recommend that you try Dahnhak Hwal-Gong. When your body is in pain there is nothing that you will appreciate more than the touch of a healing hand. Not many things will be more rewarding than knowing that you can help someone simply by laying your hands on them. The ultimate purpose of Dahnhak Hwal-Gong is to synchronize the minds of the giver and the receiver to bring about peace and joy. Hwal-Gong literally means to revive and to stimulate. It revitalizes the body and the mind; it is a "Shim-Bup", meaning "the way of the mind". Therefore, Hwal-Gong is more than just a technique. A Hwal-Gong giver must first prepare the right mindset toward the receiver. Extending a warm word with a comforting smile is also an essential aspect of Hwal-Gong.

The worst culprits in degenerating health are mindsets and lifestyles that go against life-supporting principles. If our minds wither in fear, our kidneys are weakened. If we sulk in depression, our lungs are weakened. If we burn in fury, our liver gets damaged. Aside from these internal organs, each branch of our nerves, veins, arteries; each fiber of our muscles; and every single cell in our body remembers and reacts to stress and emotional roller coasters. When these imbalanced states become chronic, 'Ki's' entry and exit points in our bodies get blocked, causing the meridians that connect our internal organs to malfunction. The root cause of many physical ailments start from here. Dahnhak Hwal-Gong is an effective method to rehabilitate balanced energy circulation by means of stimulating acupressure points and meridian channels.

It is said that ancient Korean sages comprehended the relationship between an illness and its root causes; they practiced preventing and remedying the root causes in their everyday lives. Dahnhak Hwal-Gong has adapted the wisdom of Korean ancestors to today's lifestyles. Our bodies are in their best state of health when they can be natural. The imbalance created by psychological stresses imposed upon the health of modern humans is caused by lifestyles that are disconnected from nature. This book is dedicated with our sincerest wish to help readers of this book recover their natural healthy state by using Dahnhak Hwal-Gong.

Dahn Healer School

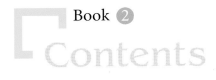

Book ❷

Contents

Preface_4

Chapter 8: *Arms and Hands*_9

1. Rubbing and Pressing the Arms_12   2. Pulling the Arms_15   3. Palm Hwal-Gong_17

Chapter 9: *Chest and Abdomen*_23

1. Chest Hwal-Gong_26   2. Smoothing the Abdomen_30   3. Relaxing Blockages in the Intestines_33   4. Pushing, Pulling, and Shaking the Abdomen_37   5. Relaxing the Lower Back_40   6. Infusing Ki_43

Chapter 10: *Front of the Legs*_49

1. Range of Motions in Ankles and Toes_52   2. Hwal-Gong on the Medial Surfaces of the Lower Extremities_56   3. Hwal-Gong on the Frontal Surfaces of the Lower Extremities_59   4. Rubbing the Knees_61   5. Hwal-Gong on the Hip Joints and Muscles of the Lower Extremities_64   6. Shaking the Lower Extremities_66

Chapter 11: *Side of the Trunk and Seated Hwal-Gong*_71

1. Wringing Muscles in the Neck and Shoulders_74   2. Pushing and Pulling the Shoulder Muscles_77   3. Relaxing the Lateral Sides of the Thighs_80   4. Hwal-Gong on the Gall Bladder Meridian in a Sideways Position_83   5. Tapping on the Gluteal Region and the Lower Extremities_88

Chapter 12: *For Advanced Practitioners*_93

1. Our Bodies: A Miniature Universe_95   2. Yin Yang, the Five Elements and the Meridians_103   3. Assesments_134   4. Strengthening and Dispersing Ki: Bo-Sah-Bup_137   5. Healing Hands Exercises for Advanced Practitioners_140

Hwal-Gong Classified by Symptoms_146

Book **1**

Preface

Chapter 1: *What is Dahnhak Hwal-Gong?*

1. Dahnhak Hwal-Gong is the Act of Giving Love   2. Seven Major Benefits of Dahnhak Hwal-Gong   3. Three Principles of Dahnhak Hwal-Gong
4. How to Touch

Chapter 2: *Preparing for Hwal-Gong*

1. Preparing for the Ideal Hwal-Gong Session   2. Hwal-Gong 1,2,3···

Chapter 3: *Turning Your Hands into Healing Hands*

1. Ki-energy and Healing Hands   2. Warm-up Exercises to Turn Your Hands into Healing Hands   3. Hand Exercises to Turn Your Hands into Healing Hands

Chapter 4: *Back Side of the Torso and Hips*

1. Relaxing the Shoulder Muscles   2. Relaxing the Shoulder Blades
3. Relaxing the Back by Rubbing and Pressing   4. Shaking while Pressing the Lower Back   5. Pressing and Rocking the Gluteal Region   6. Pressing the Spine

Chapter 5: *Back of the Legs*

1. Pressing the Soles   2. Shaking the Ankles   3. Relaxing the Calf Muscles
4. Relaxing the Posterior Sides of Thighs   5. Elevating the Knees and Pressing the Thighs   6. Rubbing and Pressing the Posterior of the Thighs

Chapter 6: *Neck and Head*

1. Pressing and Smoothing the Crown of the Head   2. Relaxing and Pressing the Neck   3. Stretching the Neck   4. Brain Hwal-Gong

Chapter 7: *Face*

1. Facial Massage   2. Facial Acupressure   3. Releasing the Jaw Joints (TMJ)

Hwal-Gong Classified by Symptoms

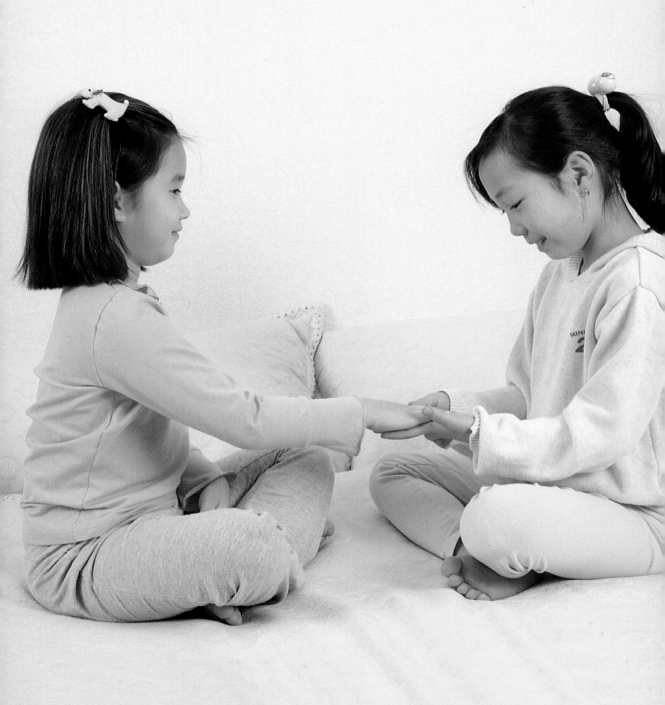

Chapter 8
Arms and Hands

1. Rubbing and Pressing the Arms
2. Pulling the Arms
3. Palm Hwal-Gong

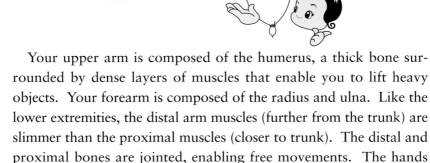

The largest area in the motor cortex of your brain is assigned to your hand coordination. Hwal-Gong on hands and arms enhances not only your motor cortex, but also your immune system. It also improves hormonal functions.

Hand Hwal-Gong will make you smarter, too.

Your upper arm is composed of the humerus, a thick bone surrounded by dense layers of muscles that enable you to lift heavy objects. Your forearm is composed of the radius and ulna. Like the lower extremities, the distal arm muscles (further from the trunk) are slimmer than the proximal muscles (closer to trunk). The distal and proximal bones are jointed, enabling free movements. The hands and arms are pathways for many nerves and meridian channels. Pericardium, Large Intestine, Heart, Small Intestine, and Lung Meridians pass along the arms. Hands and feet are complete reflexive correspondents the internal organs and have an intimate relationships with how the entire body functions.

Health diagnoses through examination of the hands, face, ears and feet are parts of a well-developed, ancient healing art. Reflexology–working on the feet and hands to affect the whole body–has a history of over 2000 years. This method is undergoing continuous scientific research and development all over the world.

Arm Hwal-Gong requires careful control in the amount of pressure applied. If an area is sensitive to strong pressure, apply pressure that is more moderate. Ask for verbal feedback from your receiver about the pressure and continually observe his/her facial expressions for signs of discomfort.

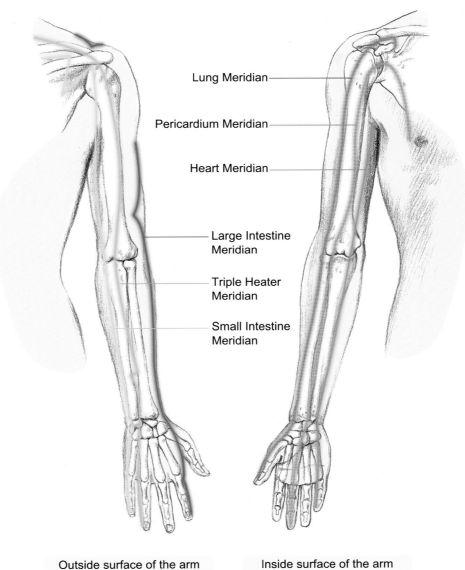

Lung Meridian

Pericardium Meridian

Heart Meridian

Large Intestine Meridian

Triple Heater Meridian

Small Intestine Meridian

Outside surface of the arm

Inside surface of the arm

Meridian channels in the upper extremities

1. Rubbing and Pressing the Arms

Hwal-Gong Techniques

Massaging with hands, rubbing to release tension

Benefits

Stimulates the meridians in the arms to improve circulation in the entire body.

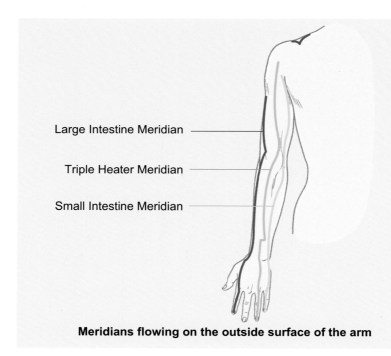

Large Intestine Meridian

Triple Heater Meridian

Small Intestine Meridian

Meridians flowing on the outside surface of the arm

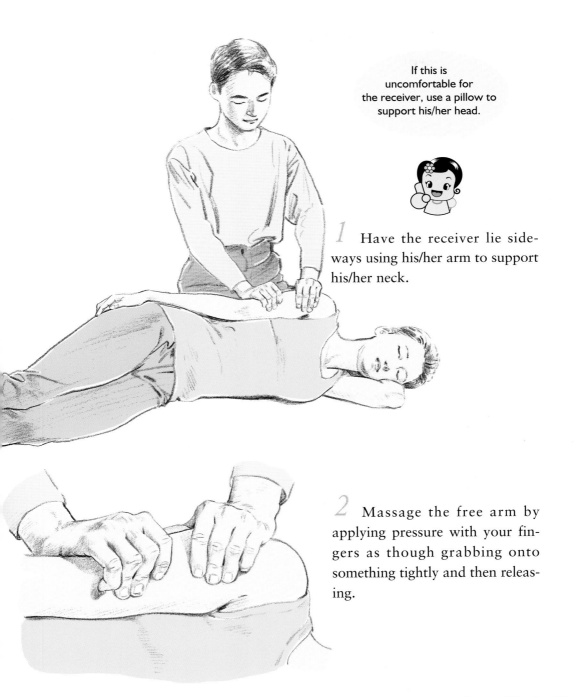

If this is uncomfortable for the receiver, use a pillow to support his/her head.

1 Have the receiver lie sideways using his/her arm to support his/her neck.

2 Massage the free arm by applying pressure with your fingers as though grabbing onto something tightly and then releasing.

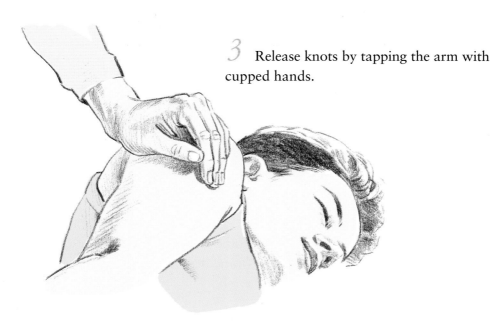

3 Release knots by tapping the arm with cupped hands.

4 Wrap your hands around the arm and shake it fast to release tension.

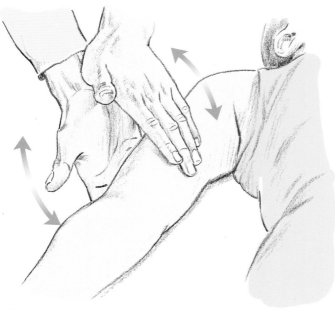

2. Pulling the Arms

Hwal-Gong Technique

Pulling the arms

Benefits

Relieves chest pain, shoulder pain, and frozen shoulders.

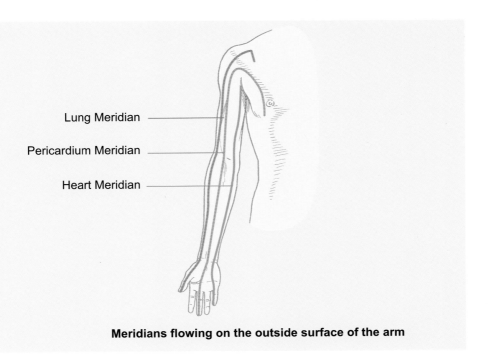

Lung Meridian

Pericardium Meridian

Heart Meridian

Meridians flowing on the outside surface of the arm

1 Have the receiver lie face up. Kneel or sit comfortably by the receiver's head.

2 Hold the receiver's wrists. Synchronize your breathing, and gradually pull upward. Pull about 60-70° up from the floor.

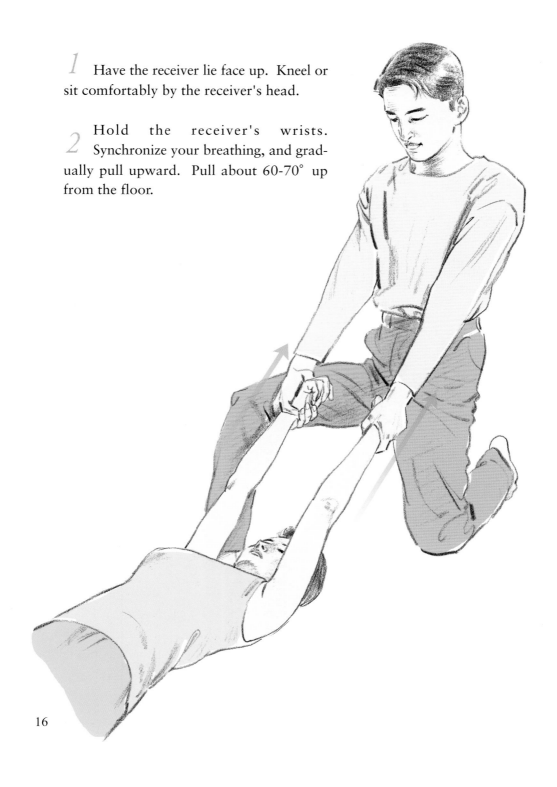

16

3. Palm Hwal-Gong

 Hwal-Gong Techniques

Pressing with thumbs, pushing

 Benefits

Relieves tension and calms the nerves. Good for relieving fatigue and all hand reflexes.

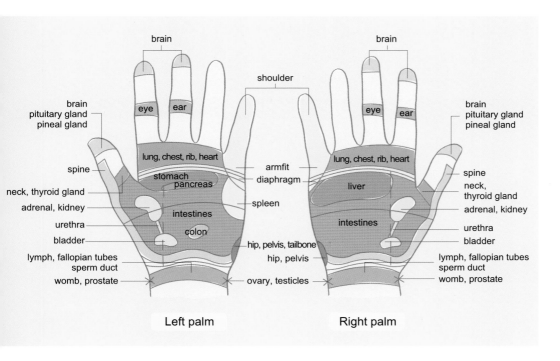

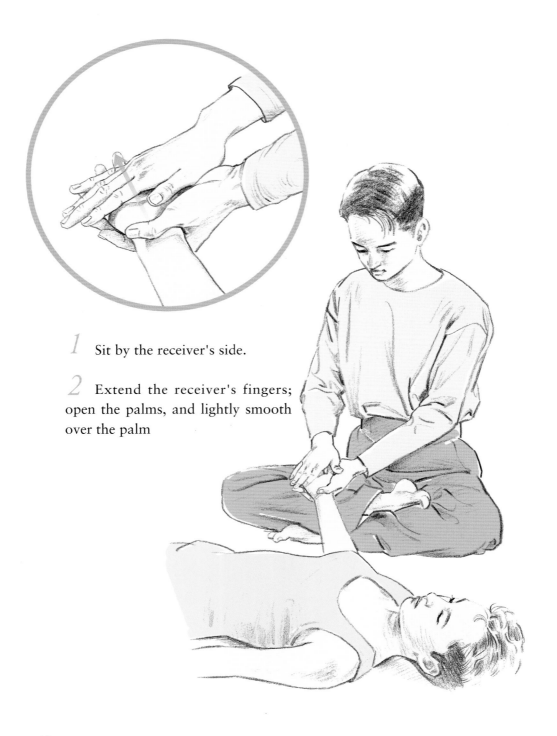

1 Sit by the receiver's side.

2 Extend the receiver's fingers;
open the palms, and lightly smooth
over the palm

18

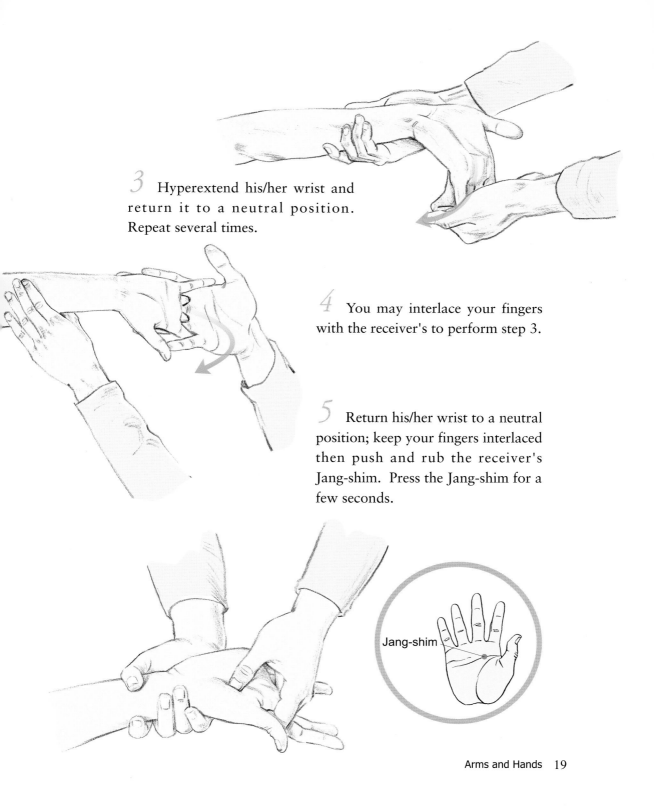

3 Hyperextend his/her wrist and return it to a neutral position. Repeat several times.

4 You may interlace your fingers with the receiver's to perform step 3.

5 Return his/her wrist to a neutral position; keep your fingers interlaced then push and rub the receiver's Jang-shim. Press the Jang-shim for a few seconds.

Jang-shim

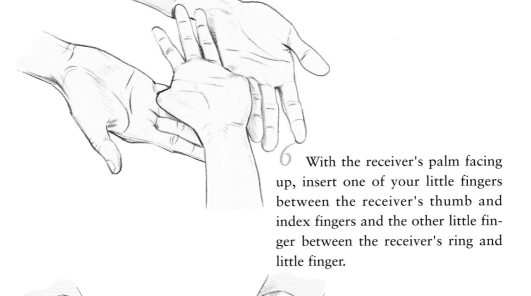

6   With the receiver's palm facing up, insert one of your little fingers between the receiver's thumb and index fingers and the other little finger between the receiver's ring and little finger.

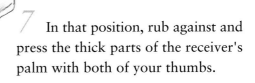

7   In that position, rub against and press the thick parts of the receiver's palm with both of your thumbs.

If the receiver feels a new sensation (such as electricity, heaviness, and pain followed by relief), when you locate an acupressure point, press that point repeatedly. The pressing and holding cycle can be as long as a breath cycle. There are many ways to accurately locate reflex points, but in general, press around the thumb and tips of fingers.

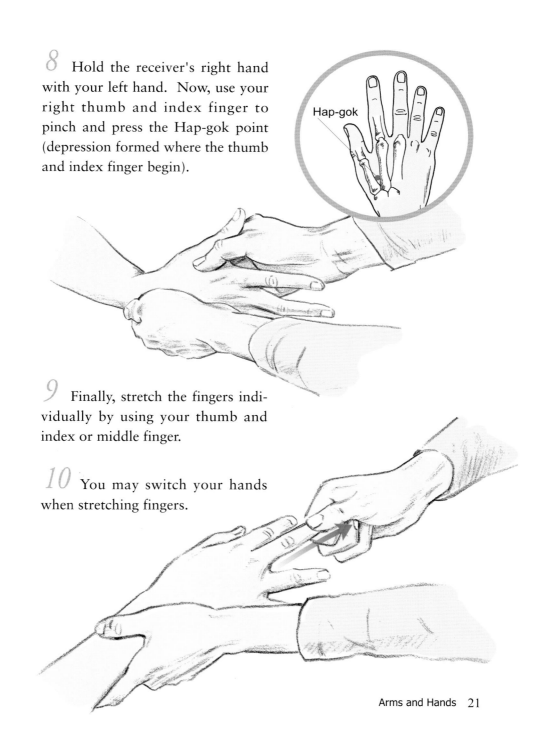

8 Hold the receiver's right hand with your left hand. Now, use your right thumb and index finger to pinch and press the Hap-gok point (depression formed where the thumb and index finger begin).

Hap-gok

9 Finally, stretch the fingers individually by using your thumb and index or middle finger.

10 You may switch your hands when stretching fingers.

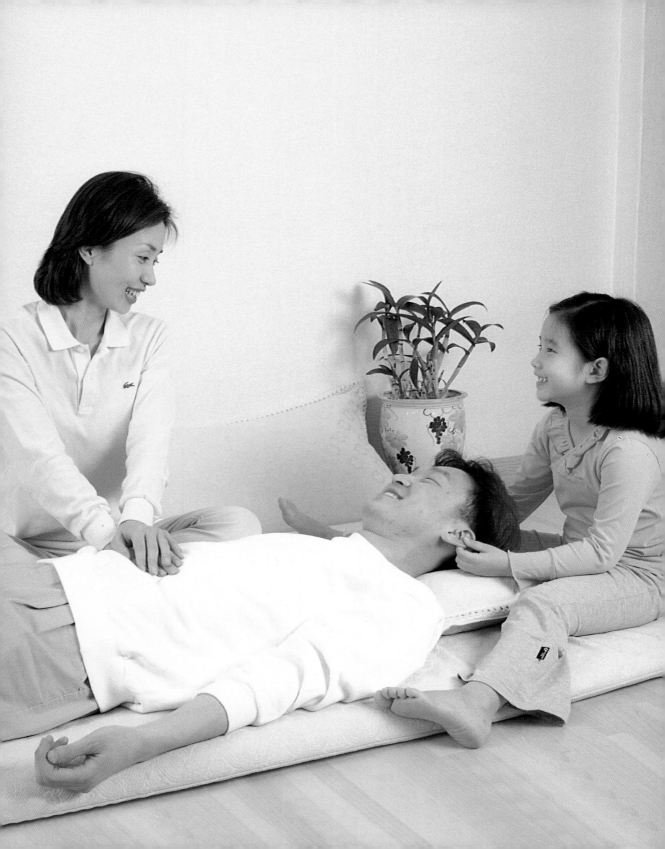

Chapter 9

Chest and Abdomen

1. Chest Hwal-Gong

2. Smoothing the Abdomen

3. Relaxing Blockages in the Intestines

4. Pushing, Pulling, and Shaking the Abdomen

5. Relaxing the Lower Back

6. Infusing Ki

When you place your hand on your chest, you can feel your heart beating. The thoracic cavity contains our vital organs, including the lungs and heart protected by the ribcage. The heart is a pump that beats about 72 cycles per minute and sends blood throughout the body. The heart supplies blood, and the lungs supply oxygen throughout the body. The thoracic cavity housing the lungs is composed of the ribcage, inter-costal muscles, and the diaphragm.

The lower area, the abdominopelvic region, contains the essential digestive organs underneath layers of cutaneous tissues and muscles. The food we eat begins a journey from our mouths to our anuses. Along the anterior of a human body flows Im-maek (Conception Meridian). The Conception Meridian brings fire energy down to Dahn-jon (an energy center in the abdominal area), and is paired with the Dok-maek (Governor Meridian) along the posterior side of the body. The Governor Meridian sends the kidneys' water energy up to the head. Excessive thoughts or anger can cause blockages in the Conception Meridian, causing poor digestion and a flushed face.

Below the navel is Lower Dahn-jon, simply called Dahn-jon. This area is central to our bodies. Therefore, good Hwal-Gong in this area can improve our bodies' systems. If someone suffers from an abdominal pain or constipation, it is better to start Hwal-Gong from his/her back. Conversely, if someone suffers from a lumbago or backache, it would be better to begin Hwal-Gong from the abdominal area.

The anterior of a human body is called Yin. Hwal-Gong in this area should be performed softly and delicately. The giver and receiver should synchronize their breathing, and the giver should carefully observe the receiver's facial expressions. It is important you perform Hwal-Gong on Dahn-jon for the purpose of increasing energy. Hwal-Gong on the chest and the solar plexus should be performed while in a calm and peaceful state of mind.

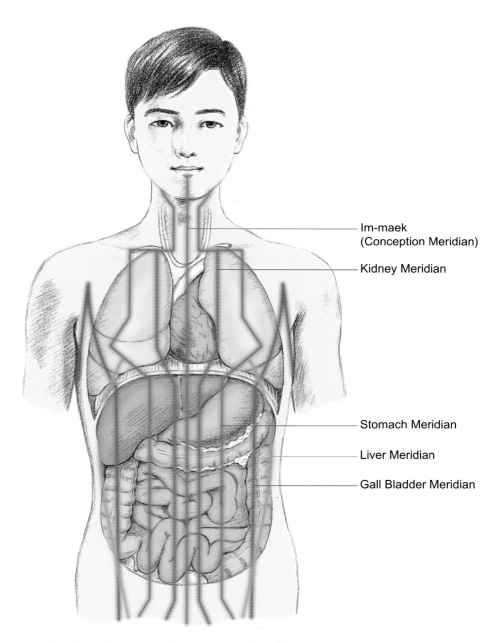

Im-maek
(Conception Meridian)

Kidney Meridian

Stomach Meridian

Liver Meridian

Gall Bladder Meridian

Meridians flowing on the anterior side of the body

1. Chest Hwal-Gong

Hwal-Gong Technique

Pressing with thumbs and palms

Benefits

Relieve anxiety, nervousness, depression, indigestion, peptic disorders, headaches, bronchitis, and chest pains.

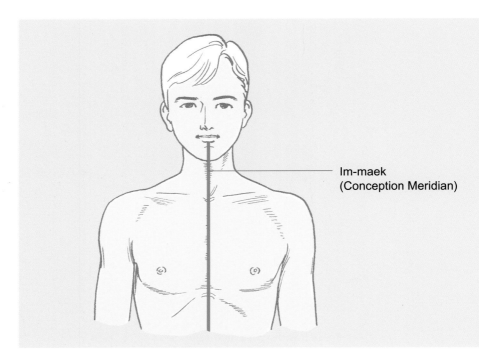

Im-maek
(Conception Meridian)

This is great in
treating depression or anger
instigated by a shock or
an emotionally traumatic event.

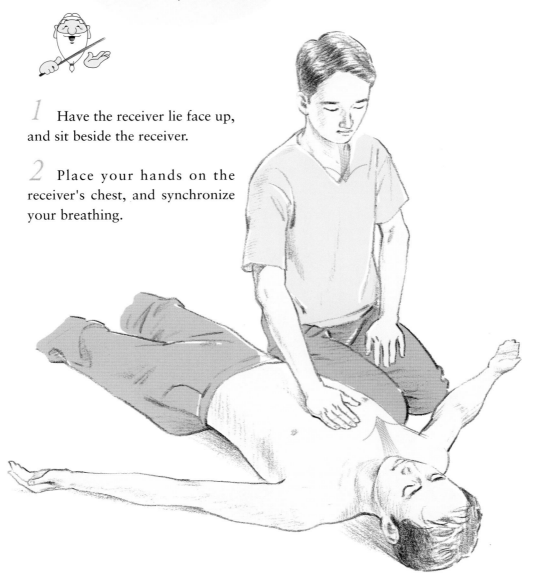

1 Have the receiver lie face up,
and sit beside the receiver.

2 Place your hands on the
receiver's chest, and synchronize
your breathing.

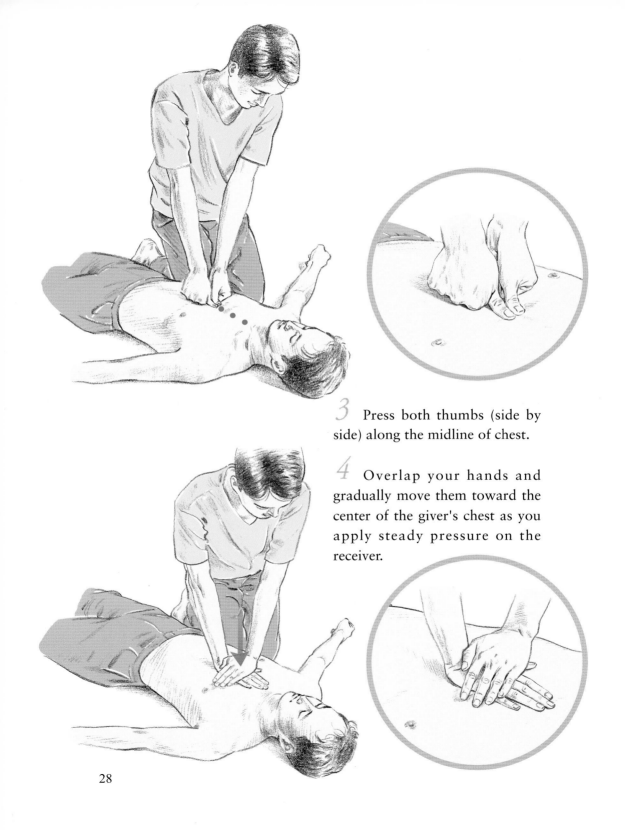

3 Press both thumbs (side by side) along the midline of chest.

4 Overlap your hands and gradually move them toward the center of the giver's chest as you apply steady pressure on the receiver.

28

If the exchange of energy between the giver and receiver is well-established, move on to the next step.

1 Place your hands on the center of the receiver's chest. Have the receiver exhale through his/her mouth. Visualize the negative energy leaving through his/her chest.

2 If you feel the energy leaving the chest, smooth down in the direction of the abdomen.

3 Place your hands on the receiver's chest, and visualize fresh energy entering his/her chest.

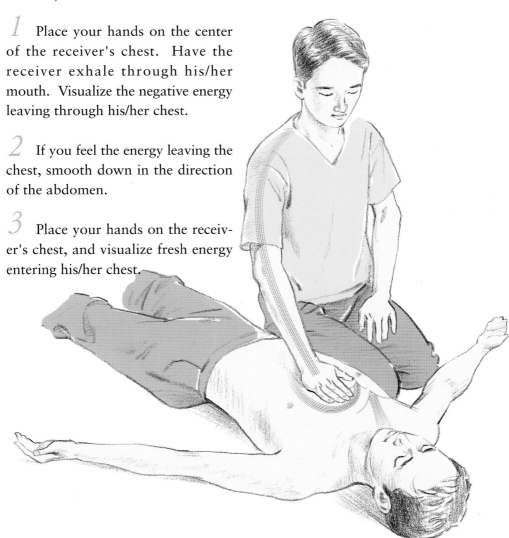

Chest and Abdomen 29

2. Smoothing the Abdomen

 Hwal-Gong Technique

Smoothing

 Benefits

Relieves abdominal cramps, diarrhea, constipation, dysentery, menstrual cramps, and uteritis.

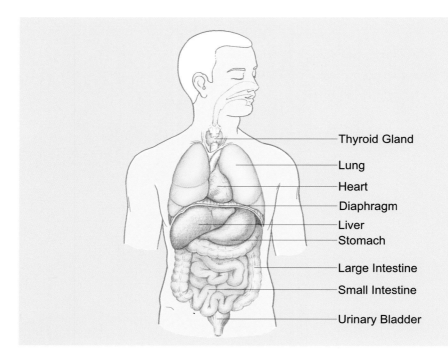

Thyroid Gland

Lung

Heart

Diaphragm

Liver

Stomach

Large Intestine

Small Intestine

Urinary Bladder

Merely laying on
your hands alone can have enough
healing effect to initiate healing signs in
the receiver, like loosening of the
intestines, burping,
or gastric sounds.

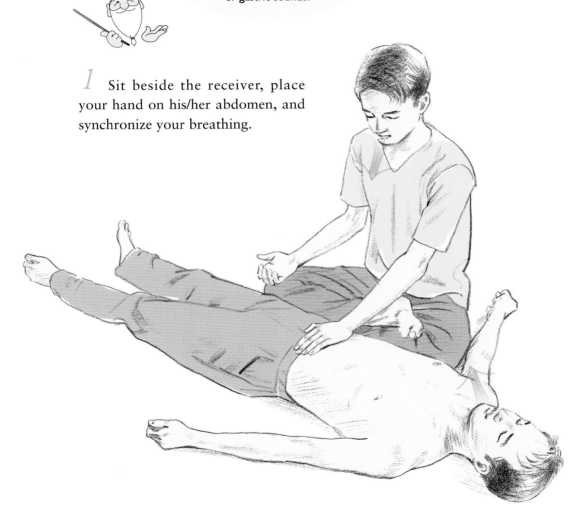

1   Sit beside the receiver, place your hand on his/her abdomen, and synchronize your breathing.

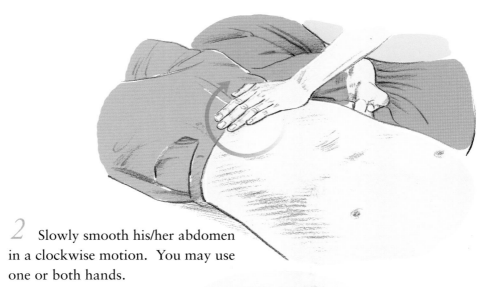

2   Slowly smooth his/her abdomen in a clockwise motion. You may use one or both hands.

This motion is in the direction of Ki flow. This is also in the same direction that the intestines lie.

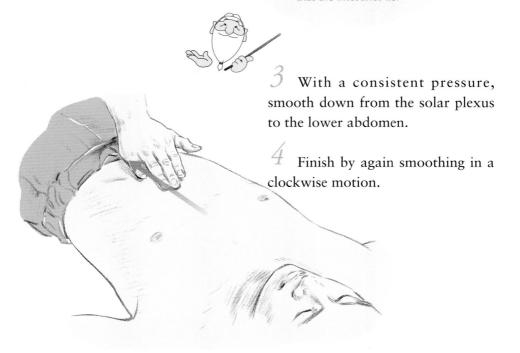

3   With a consistent pressure, smooth down from the solar plexus to the lower abdomen.

4   Finish by again smoothing in a clockwise motion.

3. Relaxing Blockages in the Intestines

Hwal-Gong Technique

Pressing with fingers

Benefits

Relieves vomiting, coughing, fatigue, inflammation of papillae (on tongue), insomnia, Raynaud's Syndrome, loss of appetite, depression, menstrual irregularity, constipation, gastric ulcer, and diarrhea.

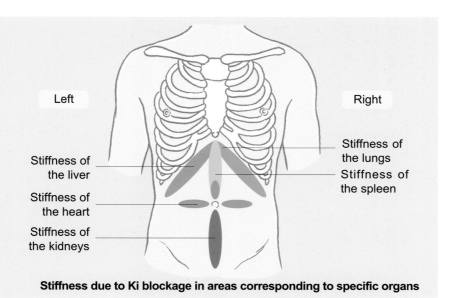

Left

Right

Stiffness of the liver

Stiffness of the lungs

Stiffness of the spleen

Stiffness of the heart

Stiffness of the kidneys

Stiffness due to Ki blockage in areas corresponding to specific organs

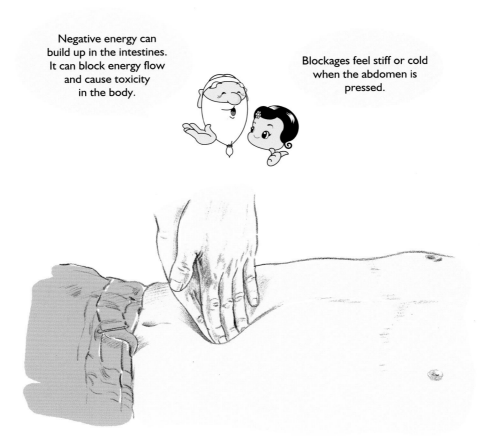

1   Have the receiver lie face up, and sit beside the receiver.

2   Release the stagnant energy in the liver. Place the tips of your right fingers (extended) below the receiver's left ribcage. Overlap your left fingertips over your right fingertips. Press down with your left hand.

3   Increase pressure with each exhalation.

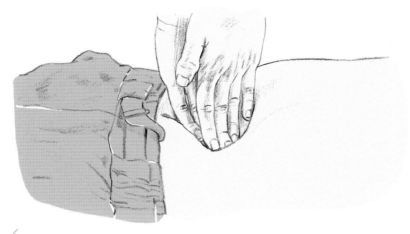

4   Release the stagnant energy in the heart. Using the same technique used for the liver, press the areas immediately above or next to the navel.

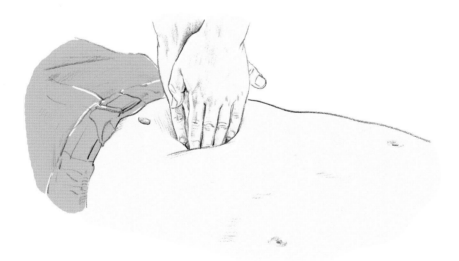

5   Stagnant energy in the spleen hardens the Joong-wahn (in between the navel and solar plexus). Use the same technique to press and release the hardness.

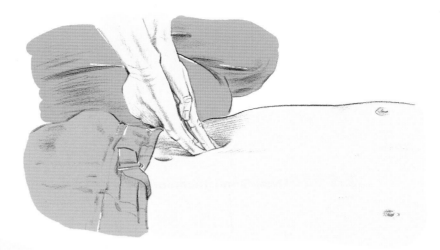

The stagnant energy in the kidneys builds along a line below the navel. Use the same method to bring relief to this area.

6 The stagnant energy in the lungs remains on the opposite side of the liver, which is below the right ribcage. Apply the same technique.

The location where energy stagnates does not always correspond with the actual organ it affects.

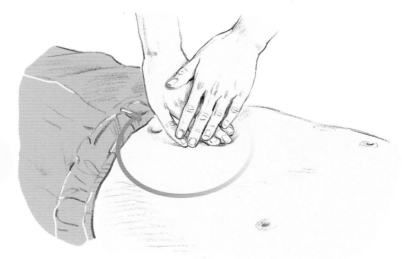

7 Finish by smoothing the abdomen in a clockwise direction.

4. Pushing, Pulling, and Shaking the Abdomen

Hwal-Gong Technique

Pushing with palms

Benefits

Relief from fatigue, indigestion, gastric ulcer, diabetes, constipation, insomnia, depression, and dysmenorrhea.

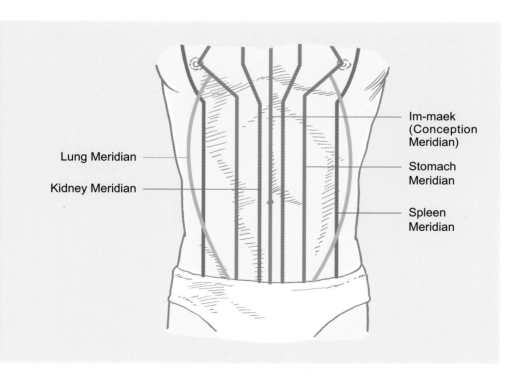

Lung Meridian

Kidney Meridian

Im-maek (Conception Meridian)

Stomach Meridian

Spleen Meridian

1 Place your hands side by side on the receiver's abdomen.

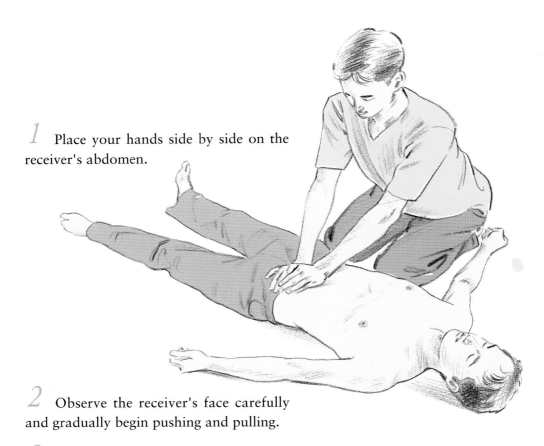

2 Observe the receiver's face carefully and gradually begin pushing and pulling.

3 Use the heels of your palms to push in a wave-like motion. Avoid rapid movements.

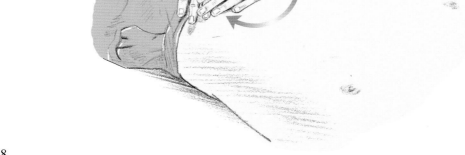

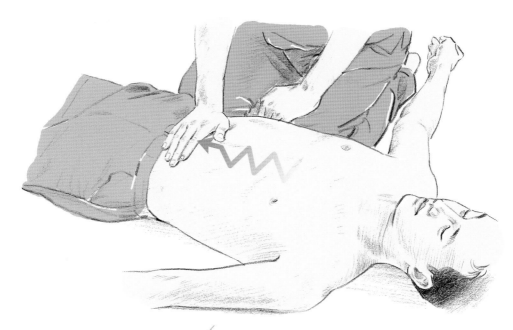

4 Starting from the solar plexus, place one hand on the receiver, and vibrate it all the way down to his/her lower abdomen.

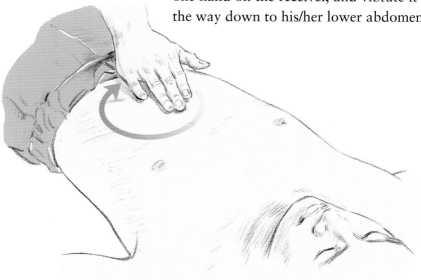

5 Finish by smoothing the abdomen in a clockwise direction.

5. Relaxing the Lower Back

Hwal-Gong Techniques

Lifting with both hands and releasing

Benefits

Relief from abdominal cramps, constipation, fatigue, indigestion, anxiety, and nervousness.

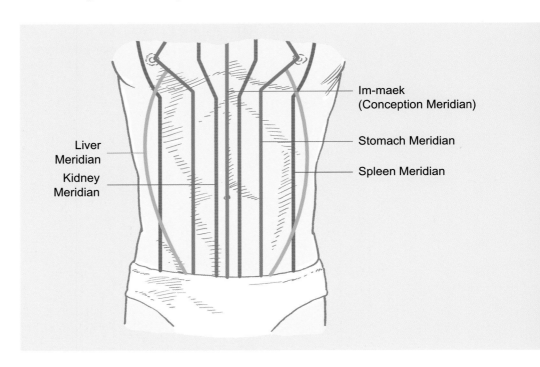

Im-maek
(Conception Meridian)

Stomach Meridian

Spleen Meridian

Liver
Meridian

Kidney
Meridian

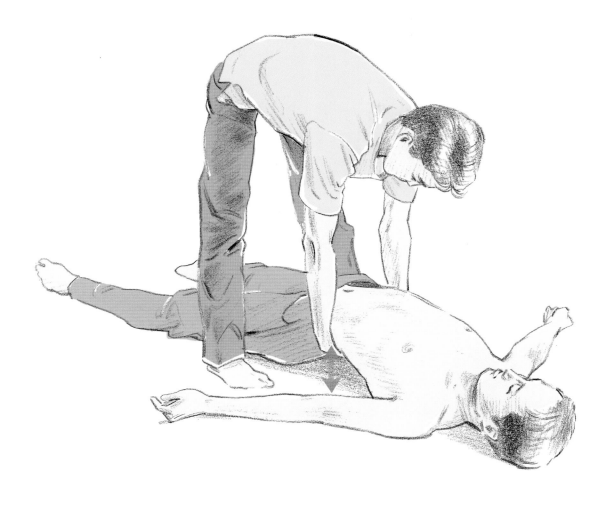

1 Have the receiver lie in a supine position. The giver's feet are at both sides of the receiver's hips. Using both hands, grasp the receiver's waist.

2 Lift the receiver's waist about 4-6 inches off the floor, and then drop it. Repeat 5-10 times.

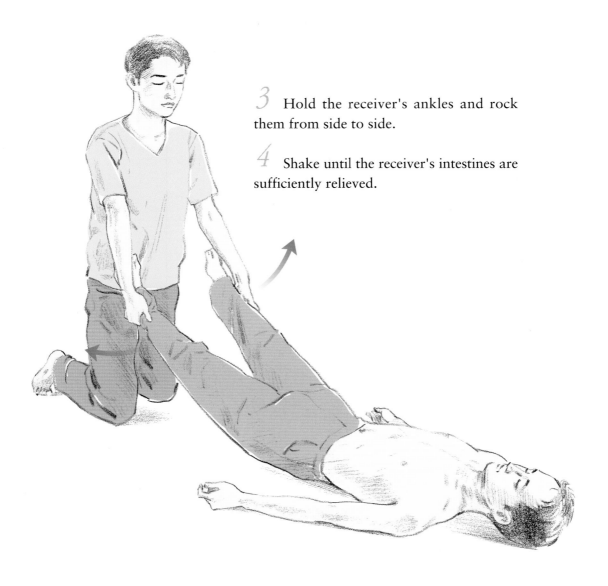

3 Hold the receiver's ankles and rock them from side to side.

4 Shake until the receiver's intestines are sufficiently relieved.

6. Infusing Ki

Hwal-Gong Technique

Infusing Ki, smoothing with palms

Benefits

Relieves vomiting, anxiety, gastritis, gastric ulcer, abdominal cramps, gastric ptosis, hypertension, diabetes, and dysmenorrhea.

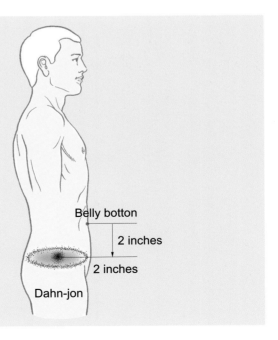

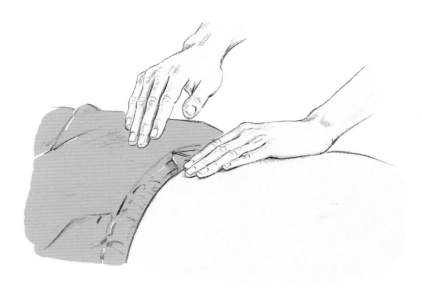

1   Sit by the receiver's side, lightly press the abdomen and smooth in a clockwise direction.

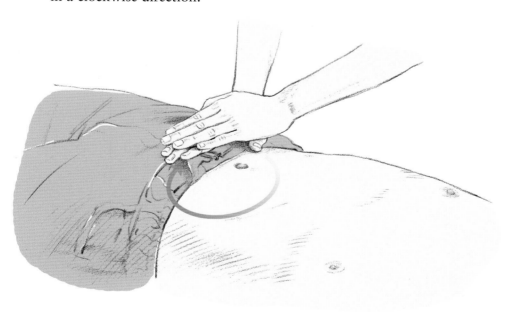

2 Place one hand on the receiver's Dahn-jon, and raise the other hand palm up.

3 Synchronize your breath with the receiver, and visualize fresh energy entering the receiver's abdomen.

4 Let the receiver know its effects by saying "Your Dahn-jon is getting hotter and hotter."

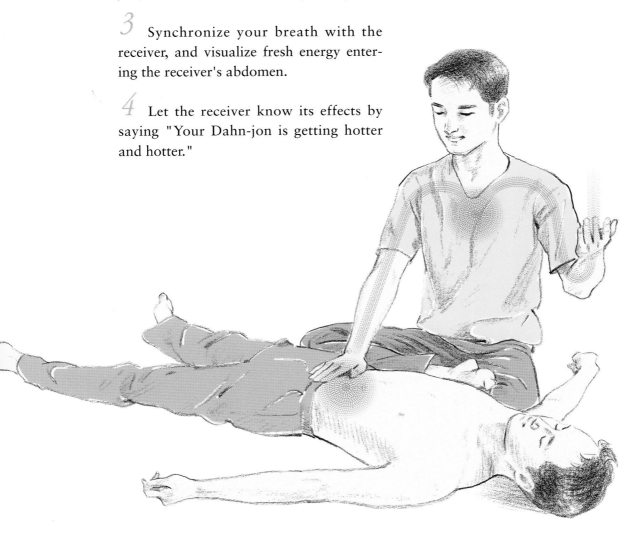

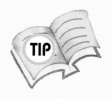 ## Diet Hwal-Gong

Heavy concentration of adipose tissues in a specific area or a weight gain in midlife are signs signaling an unnatural rhythm somewhere in the energy flow. Obesity may cause complications in people's health. When this occurs, use Hwal-Gong to restore the body's natural energy flow.

1   Have the receiver lie face up, and sit by the receiver's head. Press Gyun-jung or the border where the neck ends and the shoulders begin. Press along the shoulder line and the depression at the end known as Gyun-wu.

2   Overlap your fingers, applying pressure on your finger tips, press Joong-wahn (four fingers-width above the navel).

3   Press Chun-chu, located two fingers-width lateral to the navel.

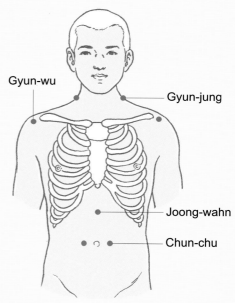

4   Extend the receiver's knees, and lightly tap the Jok-sam-ris with your fist.

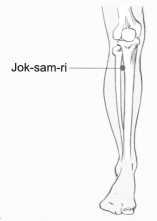

5 Have the receiver turn over on his/her abdomen, and sit by his/her side. Press along in a line about one finger-width next to the vertebral column all the way down to the hips. Tap with your fists.

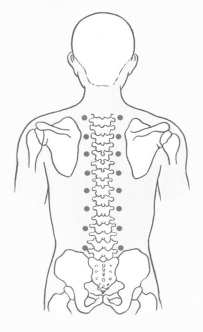

Poong-shi

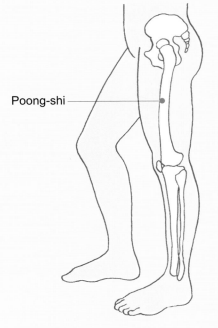

6 When the receiver is standing with his/her arms naturally resting by his/her sides, the tips of the fingers are aligned with Poong-shi on the lateral sides of the thighs. Press this point with thumb and tap with fists.

7 From the hips to the ankles, tap along the lateral line of the lower extremities with fists.

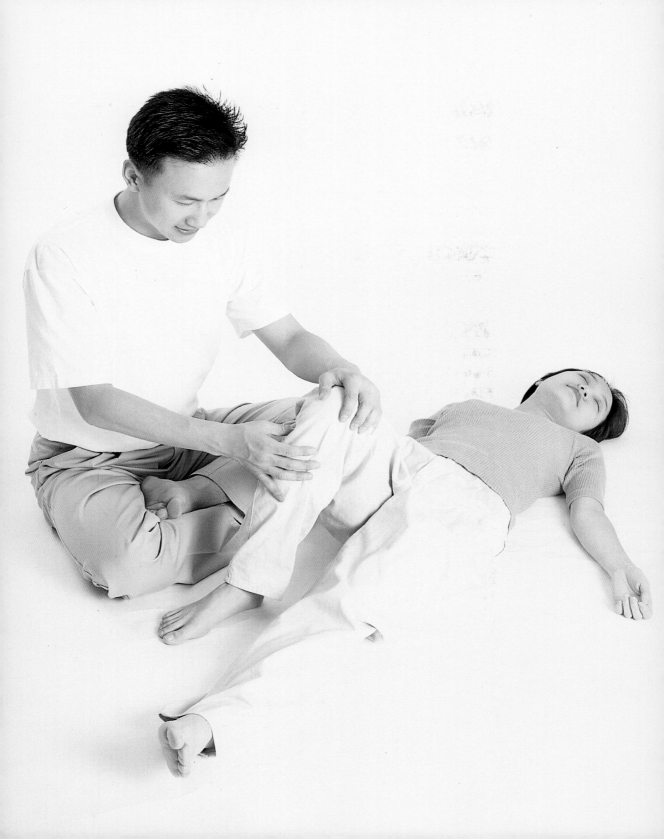

Chapter 10

Front of the Legs

1. Range of Motions in Ankles and Toes
2. Hwal-Gong on the Medial Surfaces of the Lower Extremities
3. Hwal-Gong on the Frontal Surfaces of the Lower Extremities
4. Rubbing the Knees
5. Hwal-Gong on the Hip Joints and Muscles of the Lower Extremities
6. Shaking the Lower Extremities

Our legs are like pillars for our bodies. The knees, which enable flexion and mobility, are parts of our lower extremities. Our knees are susceptible to energy stagnation, and with old age, their structures weaken and can cause much pain.

The Spleen and Liver Meridians run through the medial sides of the legs, and the Stomach Meridian runs on the lateral sides of the legs. The stomach and spleen regulate digestion and are considered "Earth" elements. Hwal-Gong on the stomach or spleen helps effective absorption of Ki from food, thereby, improving the body's overall condition and strengthening the immune system. Too much thinking and worrying steals the energy that travels from the stomach and spleen to the head. This causes nausea and a flushed face. Imbalance in the Liver Meridian weakens the spirit, and may lead to depression. On the other hand, people who are fearless and are usually confident are said to have "bigger livers."

During Hwal-Gong on the lower extremities, carefully distinguish the more muscular from the less muscular areas and adjust the pressure you apply accordingly. Practice special care around the knees.

Just like the hands
and the ears, the feet are reflexive.
Many meridian channels flow
in the feet.
A little bit of foot Hwal-Gong
can be extremely effective.

Practice simple
foot Hwal-Gong to completely
wash away a day's stress.

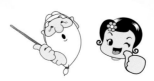

50

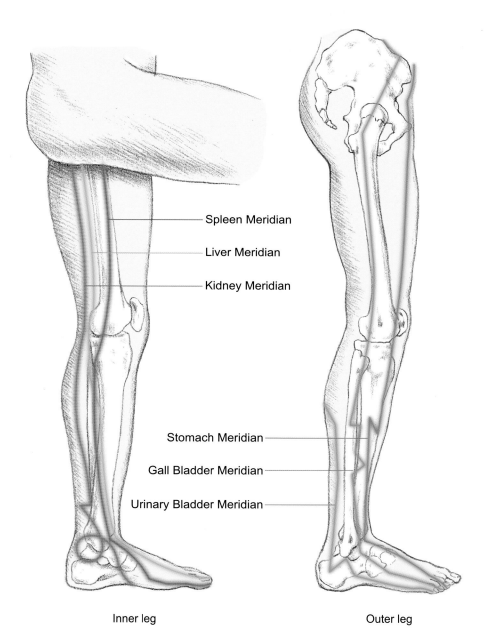

Spleen Meridian

Liver Meridian

Kidney Meridian

Stomach Meridian

Gall Bladder Meridian

Urinary Bladder Meridian

Inner leg

Outer leg

1. Range of Motions in Ankles and Toes

Hwal-Gong Technique

Pulling and stretching with fingers

Benefits

Stimulates various meridians, relieves headaches, arthritis, inflammation in the reproductive organs, bloating, and fatigue.

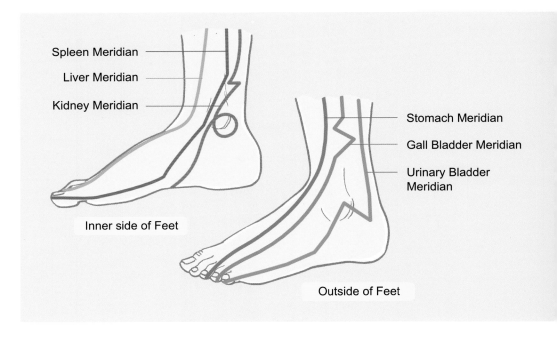

Spleen Meridian

Liver Meridian

Kidney Meridian

Stomach Meridian

Gall Bladder Meridian

Urinary Bladder Meridian

Inner side of Feet

Outside of Feet

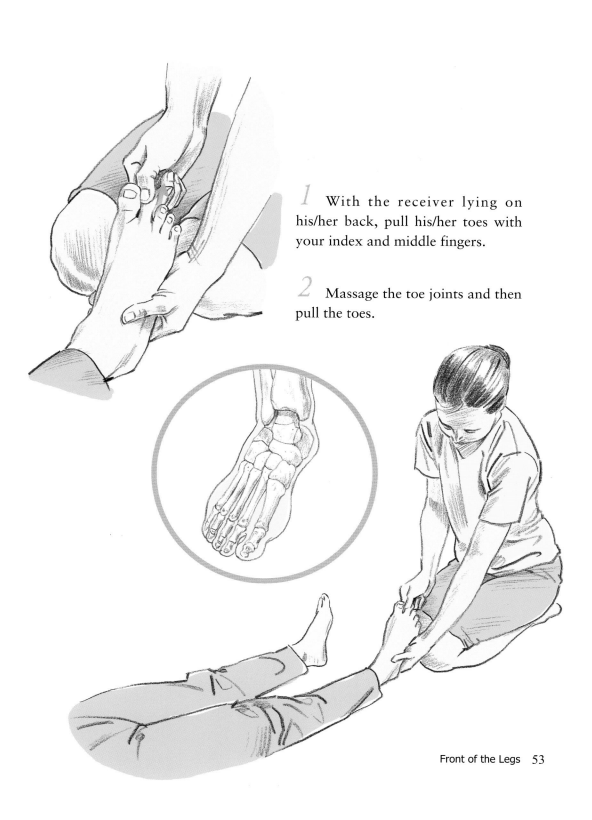

1   With the receiver lying on his/her back, pull his/her toes with your index and middle fingers.

2   Massage the toe joints and then pull the toes.

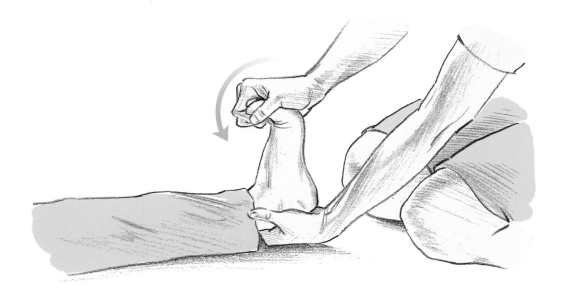

3 Support the receiver's heel with your left hand, hold the toes with your right, then push and pull the joints where the toes attach to the feet.

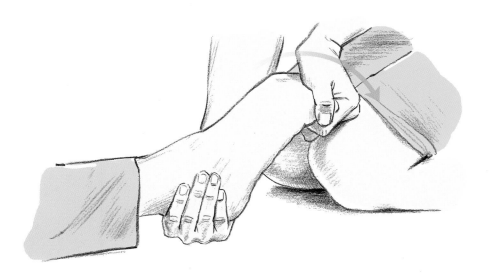

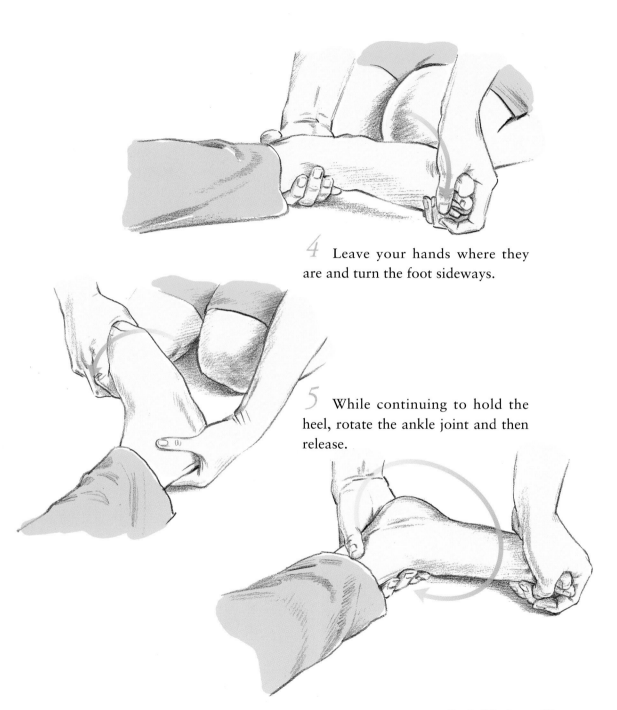

4 Leave your hands where they are and turn the foot sideways.

5 While continuing to hold the heel, rotate the ankle joint and then release.

2. Hwal-Gong on the Medial Surfaces of the Lower Extremities

Hwal-Gong Techniques

Pressing with palms, rubbing

Benefits

Relieves the Liver Meridian, leg pains, diarrhea, hepatitis, symptoms of cholecystitis, and aids recovery from eczema.

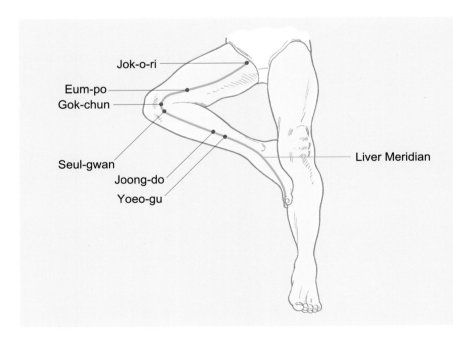

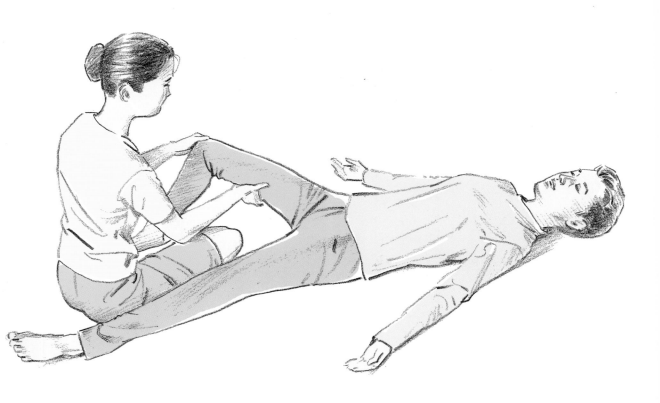

1   Have the receiver lie face up with one knee flexed while sitting by the receiver's side.

For those of you who spend most of your days sitting, this Hwal-Gong can alleviate a lot of pain.

It can also mean that your body has many blockages.

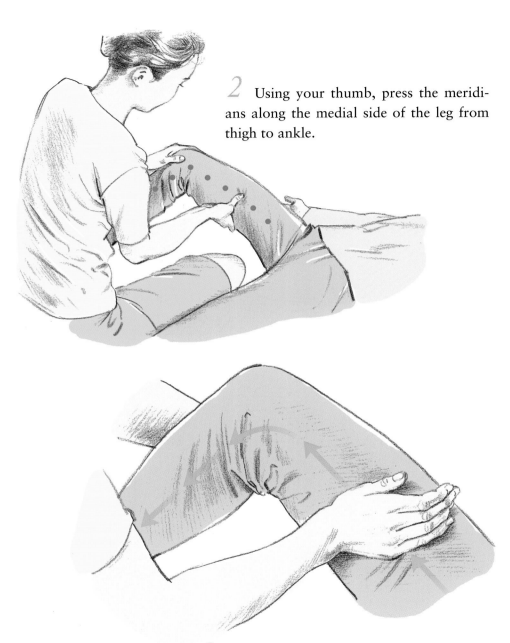

2 Using your thumb, press the meridians along the medial side of the leg from thigh to ankle.

3 Press along the same area with your palm.

4 Do the same for the other leg.

3. Hwal-Gong on the Frontal Surfaces of the Lower Extremities

Hwal-Gong Technique

Massaging

Benefits

Improves concentration and memory, relieves peptic ulcer, indigestion, gastritis, and fatigue.

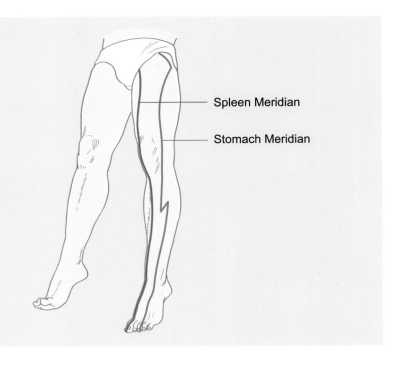

Spleen Meridian

Stomach Meridian

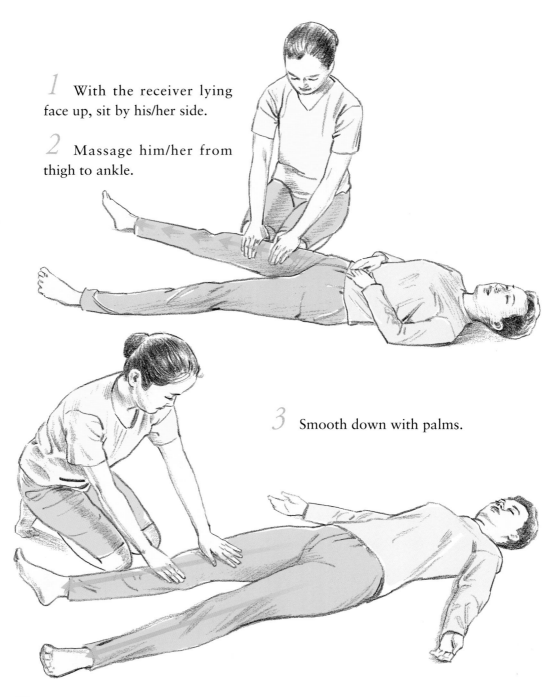

1 With the receiver lying face up, sit by his/her side.

2 Massage him/her from thigh to ankle.

3 Smooth down with palms.

60

4. Rubbing the Knees

Hwal-Gong Techniques

Rubbing with palms, pressing with thumbs

Benefits

Relieves arthritis, pain and sprain in the knees, and stimulates Stomach and Spleen Meridians.

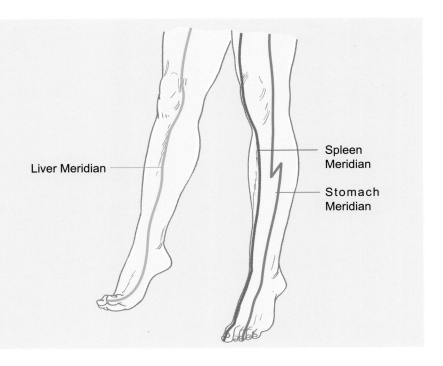

Liver Meridian

Spleen
Meridian

Stomach
Meridian

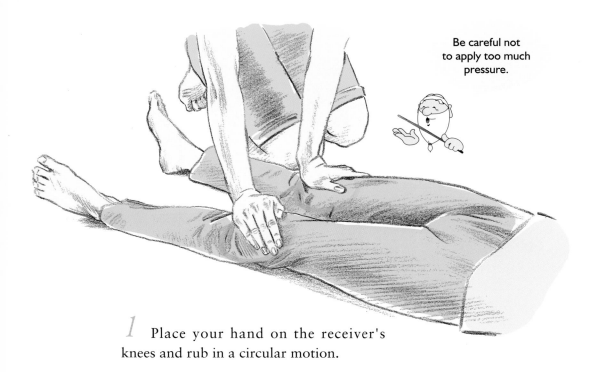

Be careful not
to apply too much
pressure.

1 Place your hand on the receiver's
knees and rub in a circular motion.

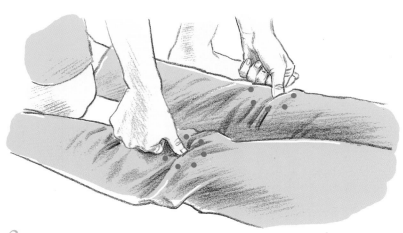

2 Press with your thumbs circling
around the knee.

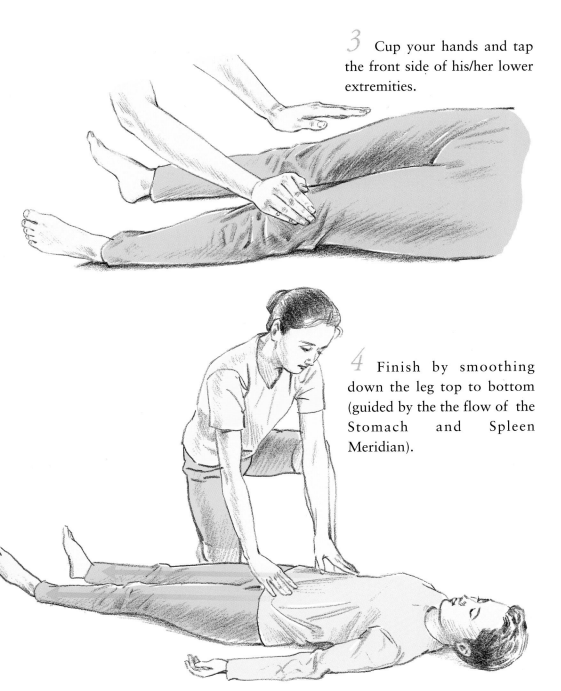

3 Cup your hands and tap the front side of his/her lower extremities.

4 Finish by smoothing down the leg top to bottom (guided by the the flow of the Stomach and Spleen Meridian).

5. Hwal-Gong on the Hip Joints and Muscles in the Lower Extremities

Hwal-Gong Techniques

Pushing and rolling with hands

Benefits

Relieves muscles around the hip joints and stimulates the Spleen and Stomach Meridians.

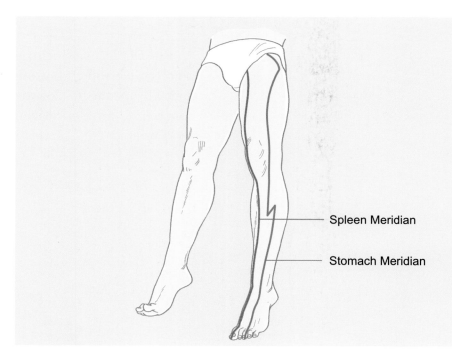

Spleen Meridian

Stomach Meridian

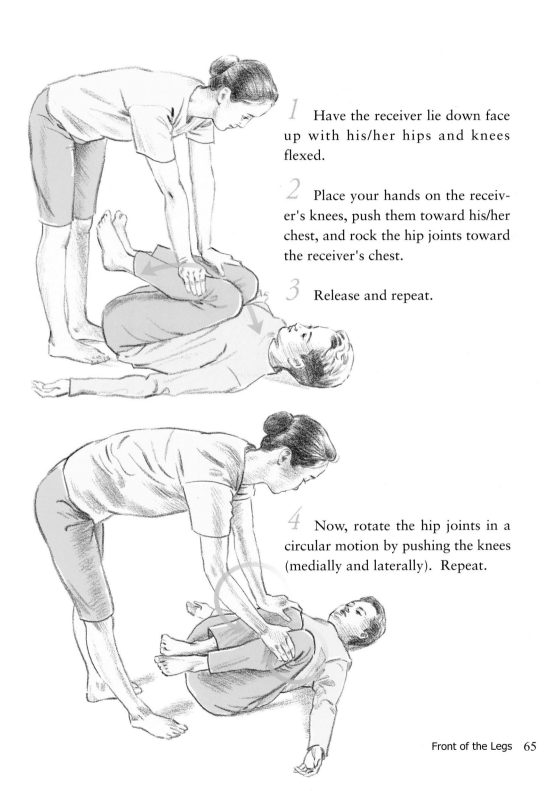

_1_ Have the receiver lie down face up with his/her hips and knees flexed.

_2_ Place your hands on the receiver's knees, push them toward his/her chest, and rock the hip joints toward the receiver's chest.

_3_ Release and repeat.

_4_ Now, rotate the hip joints in a circular motion by pushing the knees (medially and laterally). Repeat.

6. Shaking the Lower Extremities

Hwal-Gong Technique

Shaking

Benefits

Circulates stagnant blood and Ki trapped in the legs due to gravity and lack of movement. This will aid recovery from fatigue, speed circulation, and hypertension.

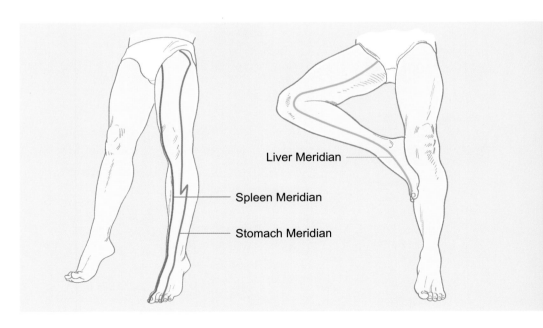

Liver Meridian

Spleen Meridian

Stomach Meridian

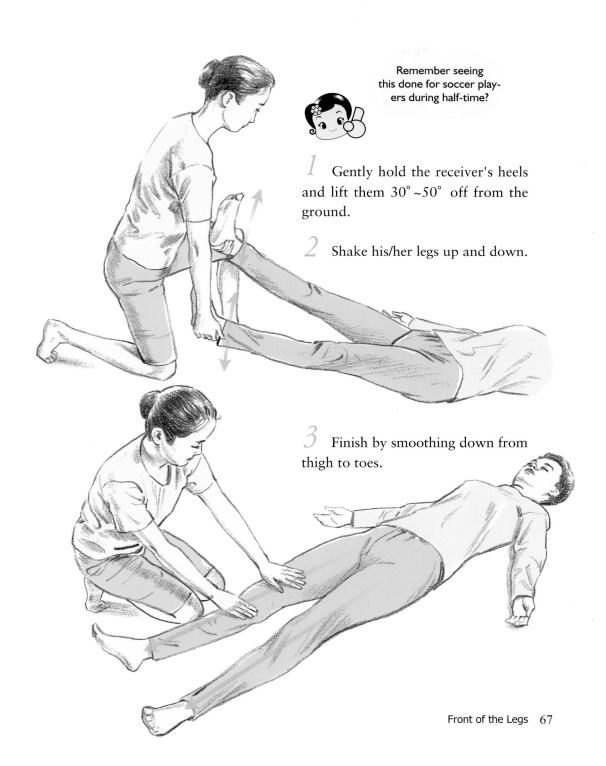

Remember seeing this done for soccer players during half-time?

1 Gently hold the receiver's heels and lift them 30°~50° off from the ground.

2 Shake his/her legs up and down.

3 Finish by smoothing down from thigh to toes.

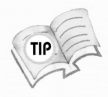

Pregnancy Hwal-Gong

Pregnancy Hwal-Gong can be divided into first, second, and third trimesters. Have the receiver lie sideways and perform Hwal-Gong on her back. Do not apply deep pressure.

First Trimester Hwal-Gong

The first and second months of pregnancy can easily go unnoticed. Therefore, when there is a possibility that the receiver may be pregnant, practice caution. During the second month, the embryo's Gall Bladder Meridian begins to form, the heart, and the brain develop rapidly. From the third month on, the kidneys develop, and in the fourth month, the Triple Heater Meridian develops.

Have the receiver lie sideways, and perform Hwal-Gong from shoulder to legs along the Urinary Bladder Meridian to increase energy in the Kidney Meridian. The receiver and giver may visualize the healthy development of the unborn child. This will help energy be transfered to the child. Avoid applying Hwal-Gong on the Gall Bladder Meridian on top of the shoulders and the Yin Meridians on the medial sides of the legs.

Second Trimester Hwal-Gong

The fetus in its fifth month of gestation has an egg-sized head that is about 1/3 the size of its entire body. Energy begins to build up in the Spleen Meridian; steady growth of this meridian will result in the child's tendencies to have deep thoughts. During the sixth month, the bones are aligned and the auditory senses develop. In the seventh month, there is sufficient development of the cerebral cortex as well as the Lung Meridian. During this time, practice a lot of Brain Hwal-Gong and visualize growth of the fetus's brain. Hwal-Gong on the Urinary Bladder Meridian is important as always.

Third Trimester Hwal-Gong

In the eighth month, lungs and large intestine are formed and the auditory senses are fully developed. In the ninth month, energy begins to build up in the Kidney Meridian. In the tenth month, the Urinary Bladder Meridian is finally energized, thereby completing the energy build-up in all Five Jangs (Viscera) and Six Bus (Organs). Congratulate the baby for having endured the months of gestation by preparing for its beginning in this world. In the postpartum phase, the mother may suffer from pains especially in the lower back and hip areas. Have her rest on her stomach, and apply Hwal-Gong on these areas.

Infant Hwal-Gong

During the first month, the newborn cannot distinguish himself/herself from the outside world. However, when the soft spot on the crown of the head (Baek-hwae) begins to close, the baby begins to decipher color and sound and becomes more responsive to external stimuli. From this point on, the baby's cries are clearly distinct based on the reasons for the cries (hunger, tiredness, or illness). Don't automatically react to the baby's cry by feeding or putting him/her to sleep. Instead, apply appropriate Hwal-Gong to prevent illnesses and ensure healthy growth.

Infants learn about love and the external world by touching. Hwal-Gong has positive emotional effects for the baby who cannot yet talk. In addition, frequent Hwal-Gong while changing diapers can prevent rash without resorting to medication. Avoid pressing or applying intense stimulation. The best methods are gentle touches and smoothing down with palms.

1. Smooth down from the chest to the abdomen. Smooth slowly and gradually. Smooth the back of the baby and the arms as well.
2. If the baby startles easily or is generally weak, smooth in both upward and medial directions.
3. Gently massage the arms and the legs. Smooth the chest and abdomen in a clockwise motion.
4. Lay the baby prone and smooth from bottom up, and from lateral to medial (bringing your hands together in the center).
5. Very lightly, press the baby's entire face with your thumb.

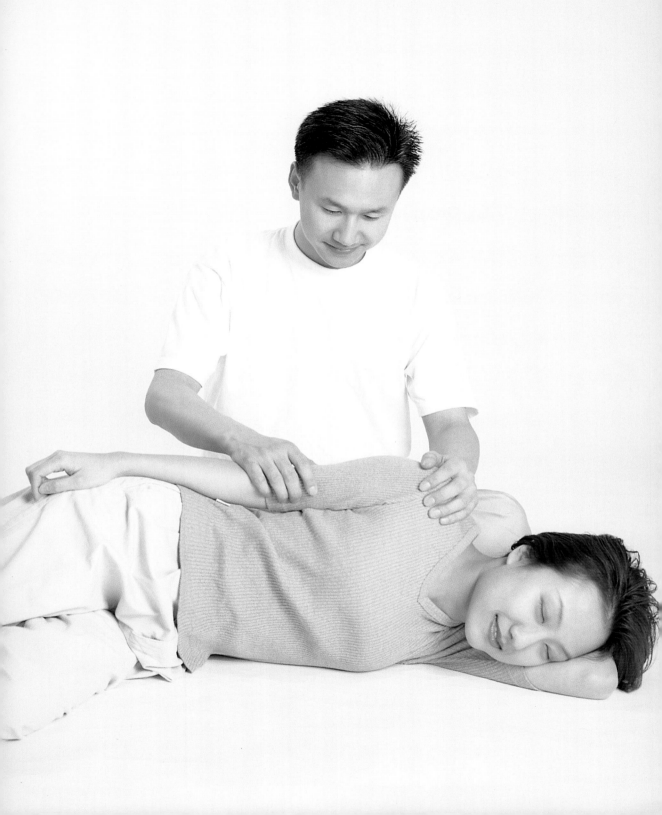

Chapter 11

Side of the Trunk and Seated Hwal-Gong

1. Wringing Muscles in Neck and Shoulders
2. Pushing and Pulling the Shoulder Muscles
3. Relaxing the Lateral Sides of the Thighs
4. Hwal-Gong on the Gall Bladder Meridian in a Sideways Position
5. Foot Tapping on the Gluteal Region and the Lower Extremities

The side of the body can be divided into two parts; one from head to toes (the axial portion), and the other from head to fingers (the appendicular portion). From head to toes runs the Gall Bladder Meridian which is paired with the Liver Meridian that runs on the medial aspect of the leg. The liver is an irreplaceable organ that performs various functions. Most importantly, it carries on its endless task of detoxifying the body.

The Gall Bladder helps digestion. Weaknesses in the liver and the Gall Bladder makes one susceptible to fatigue, anger (due to poor digestion), fear, loss of will power, and may cause dry lips.

The sides of the arms lie pathways for the Triple Heater Meridian which aids the kidneys. Blockage in this meridian leads to fever or illness in the ears and the eyes.

When beginning Hwal-Gong on the side of the body, caution the receiver not to turn abruptly. Softly massage the side of the body and support the back of the body with both hands. Then the receiver will naturally turn to his/her side.

The benefit to a seated position is that it enables many Hwal-Gong techniques that are awkward or difficult to do in a recumbent position. This position is often used for performing Hwal-Gong on the head, neck, and shoulders. It is recommended to begin this Hwal-Gong with a gradual release of the shoulders in a seated Hwal-Gong position.

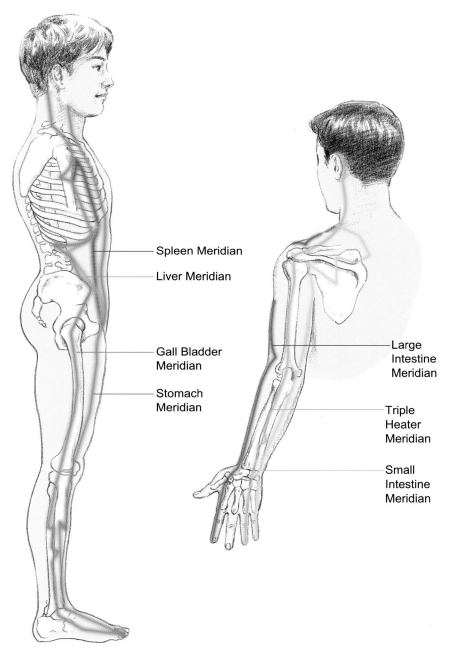

Spleen Meridian

Liver Meridian

Gall Bladder Meridian

Stomach Meridian

Large Intestine Meridian

Triple Heater Meridian

Small Intestine Meridian

Meridians that run along the side of the body

1. Wringing Muscles in the Neck and Shoulders

Hwal-Gong Technique

Wringing with both hands

Benefits

Relieves shoulder pains from old age, fatigue, headaches, and indigestion.

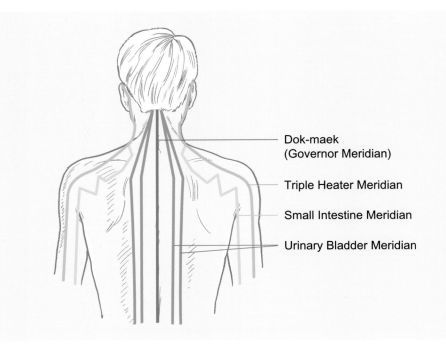

Dok-maek
(Governor Meridian)

Triple Heater Meridian

Small Intestine Meridian

Urinary Bladder Meridian

1 Have the receiver sit in the full or half lotus position or sit comfortably with legs crossed.

2 Kneel down behind the receiver, and instruct the receiver to flex his/her neck slightly. Clasp your hands behind the receiver's neck.

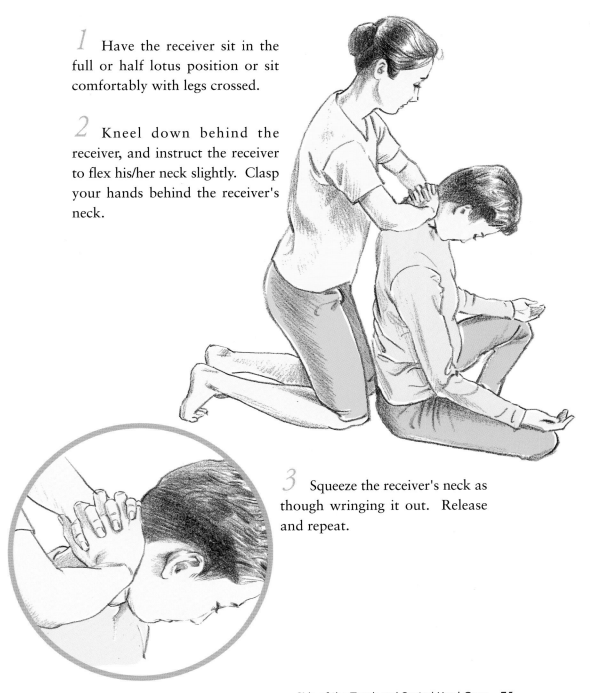

3 Squeeze the receiver's neck as though wringing it out. Release and repeat.

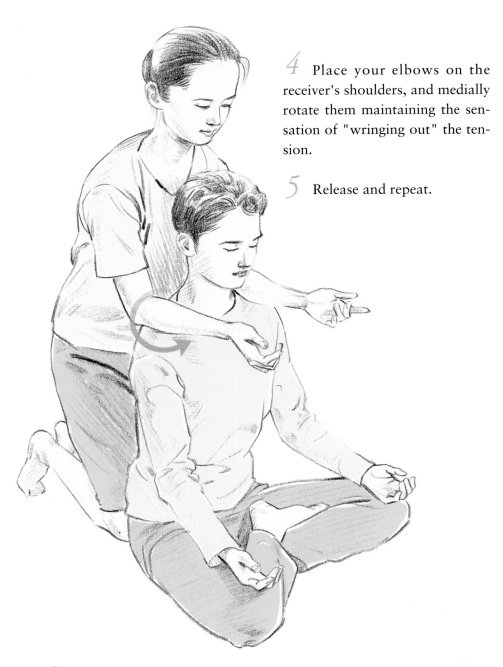

4　Place your elbows on the receiver's shoulders, and medially rotate them maintaining the sensation of "wringing out" the tension.

5　Release and repeat.

2. Pushing and Pulling the Shoulder Muscles

Hwal-Gong Techniques

Pressing with thumbs, clasping hands, and squeezeing the muscles

Benefits

Relieves fatigue, heart disease, pain in arms and shoulders

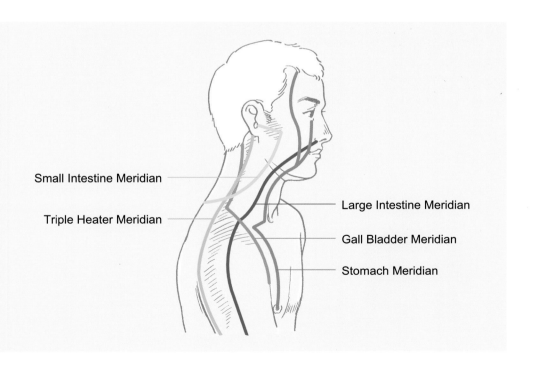

Small Intestine Meridian

Triple Heater Meridian

Large Intestine Meridian

Gall Bladder Meridian

Stomach Meridian

1 Have the receiver lie on his/her side with his/her head supported by his/her own arm. Secure your right hand on the receiver's shoulder by pressing on it, and squeeze the shoulder with your left hand.

2 With the receiver's shoulder secured by your right hand, use the left thumb to press underneath the medial border of the shoulder blades.

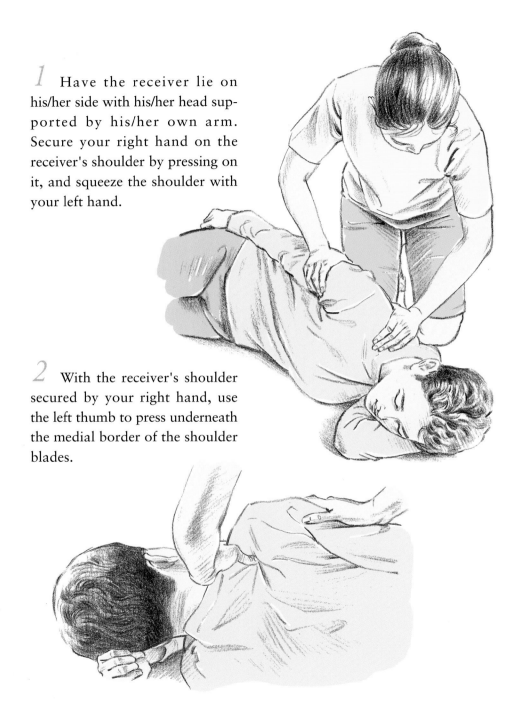

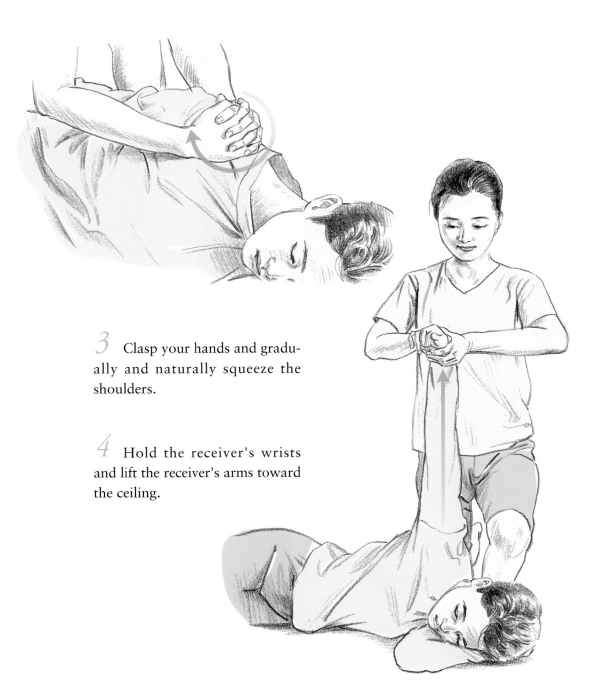

3   Clasp your hands and gradually and naturally squeeze the shoulders.

4   Hold the receiver's wrists and lift the receiver's arms toward the ceiling.

3. Releasing the Lateral sides of the Thighs

Hwal-Gong Technique

Pressing with thumbs

Benefits

Relieves neuralgia, knee arthritis, paralysis in lower extremities, and hemiplegia. If the ileofemoral joint (hip joint) is out of alignment, not only will the lower back hurt, but the internal organs will also suffer from being misplaced. This Hwal-Gong opens up the meridians and also helps realign the hip joints.

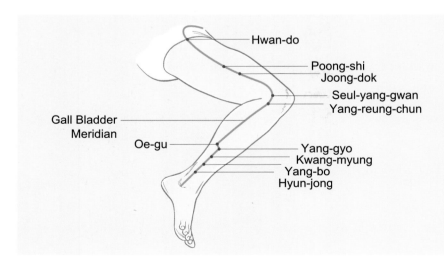

If the hip joints are not aligned properly, not only does it cause lower back pain, the organs are shifted and this can cause dysfuntion of the organs.

So you can use this technique to open the meridian channels as well as realign the hip joints.

1 Have the receiver lie in a prone position, and sit by the receiver's feet. Take the receiver's right leg and places it over the left leg (laterally rotate the thighs and flex the knees).

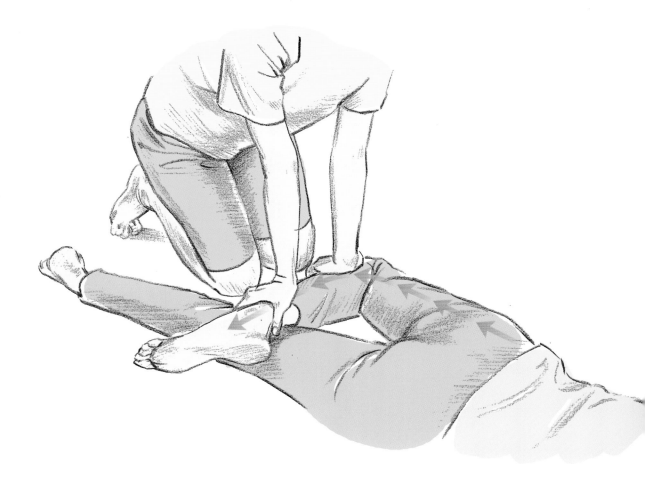

2 Stabilize the receiver's right ankle with your left hand, and compress the lateral side of the thigh to the knee and from the knee down to the ankle.

3 Repeat twice and then switch legs.

4. Hwal-Gong on the Gall Bladder Meridian in a Sideways Position

Hwal-Gong Techniques

Massaging with hands, pressing with thumbs

Benefits

Relieves constipation, indigestion, colon and stomach dysfunctions, bronchitis, pneumonia, shoulder pain, and frozen shoulders.

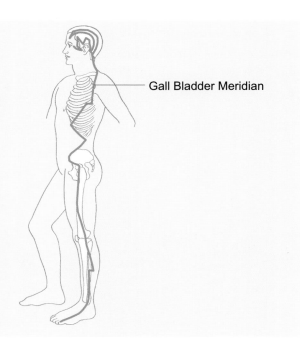

Gall Bladder Meridian

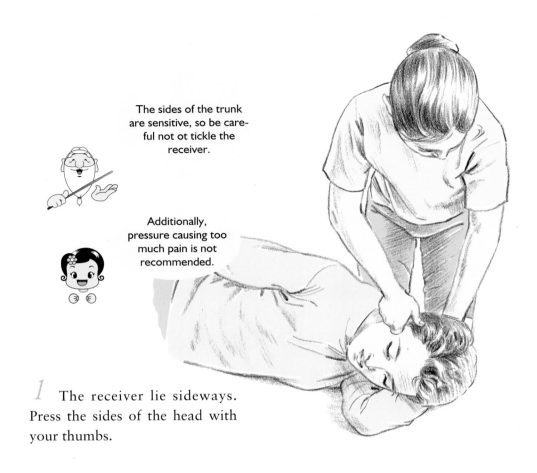

The sides of the trunk are sensitive, so be careful not ot tickle the receiver.

Additionally, pressure causing too much pain is not recommended.

1 The receiver lie sideways. Press the sides of the head with your thumbs.

2 Massage the muscle group in the back of the neck.

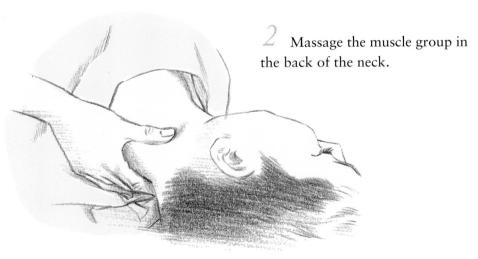

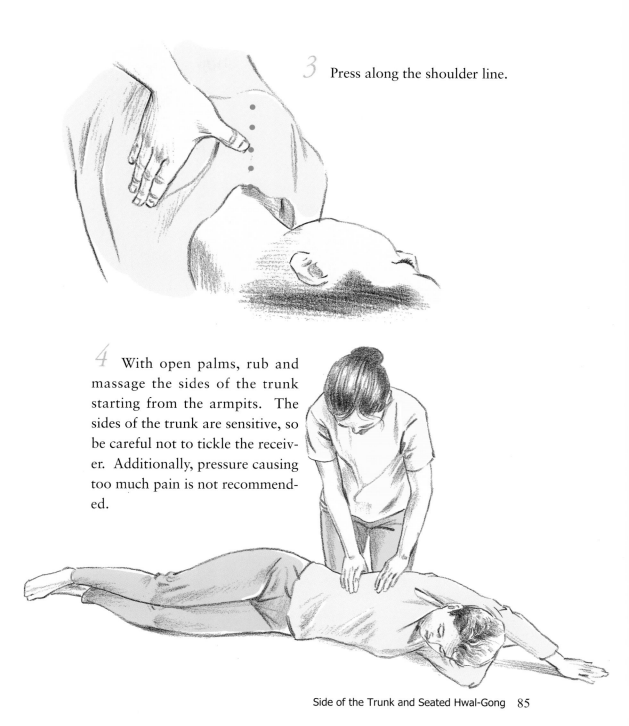

3 Press along the shoulder line.

4 With open palms, rub and massage the sides of the trunk starting from the armpits. The sides of the trunk are sensitive, so be careful not to tickle the receiver. Additionally, pressure causing too much pain is not recommended.

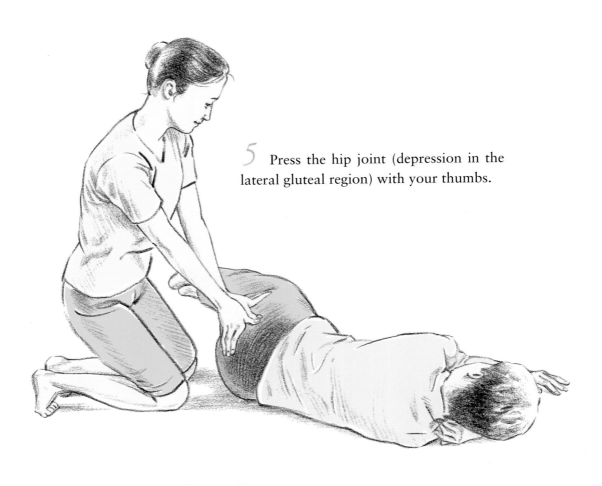

5 Press the hip joint (depression in the lateral gluteal region) with your thumbs.

You can identify
its location by a man's back
pocket button on his suit
trousers.

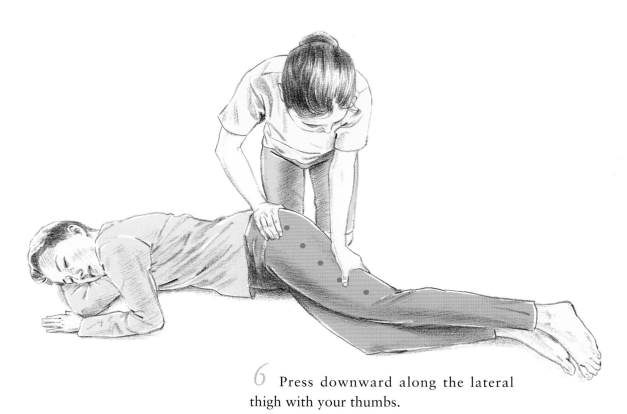

6 Press downward along the lateral thigh with your thumbs.

7 Press downward along the lower leg with your thumbs.

5. Tapping on the Gluteal Region and Lower Extremities

Hwal-Gong Technique

Tapping with fist

Benefits

Relieves sciatica, lower back pain, paralysis of lower extremities, and beriberi

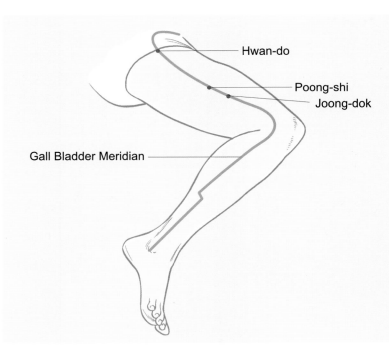

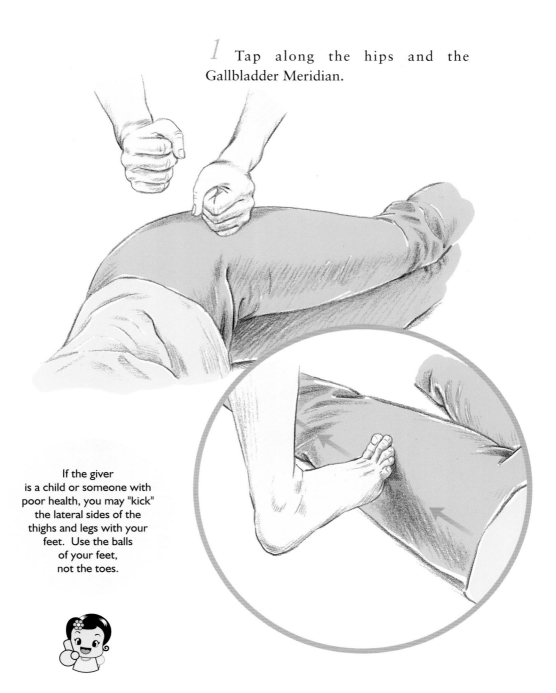

1 Tap along the hips and the Gallbladder Meridian.

If the giver is a child or someone with poor health, you may "kick" the lateral sides of the thighs and legs with your feet. Use the balls of your feet, not the toes.

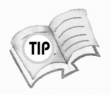

TIP

Seated Hwal-Gong

Anyone working in an office can use a good massage around noon. Massaging one another is sure to give a lift to your body and mind. It is difficult to perform Hwal-Gong on the front part of the body when someone is in a seated position. However, thorough Hwal-Gong on just the shoulders, arms, head, and palms will have excellent results.

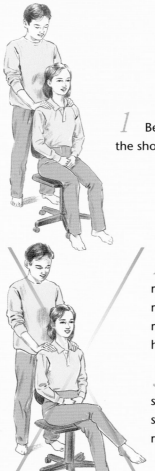

1 Begin by massaging the shoulders.

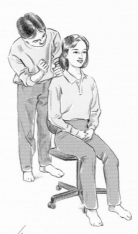

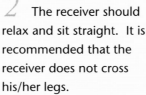

2 The receiver should relax and sit straight. It is recommended that the receiver does not cross his/her legs.

3 Hwal-Gong on the scapulas is performed the same way as when the receiver is prone.

4 When applying pressure on the receiver's back, it may be difficult to maintain consistent pressure because the receiver's body tends to be pushed forward. Instead of pressing with your thumbs, lightly tap his/her back with your palms or fists. If the receiver is weak, it is good enough to just smooth down his/her entire back.

90

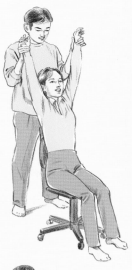

5 Lift both of the receiver's arms, and stretch them up. Effective stretching will release tension and fatigue and promote healthy energy to circulate.

Hwal-Gong in a sitting position involves some techniques used in lying positions. However, be prepared to revise the techniques to make sure that the receiver's position is balanced and that his/her body does not sway too much. Hand Hwal-Gong requires special finesse.

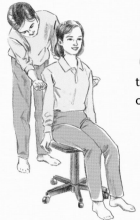

6 Return the arms to the side and tap the sides of the arms.

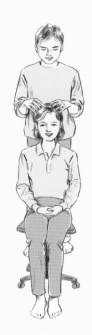

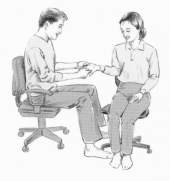

7 Now, the giver may sit and perform hand Hwal-Gong. Instead of sitting face to face, the most comfortable position for both people may be for the giver to sit facing the side of the receiver (perpendicularly to each other).

8 Get behind the receiver to tap and smooth his/her head. The receiver may rest his/her head on a headrest as you perform Brain Hwal-Gong.

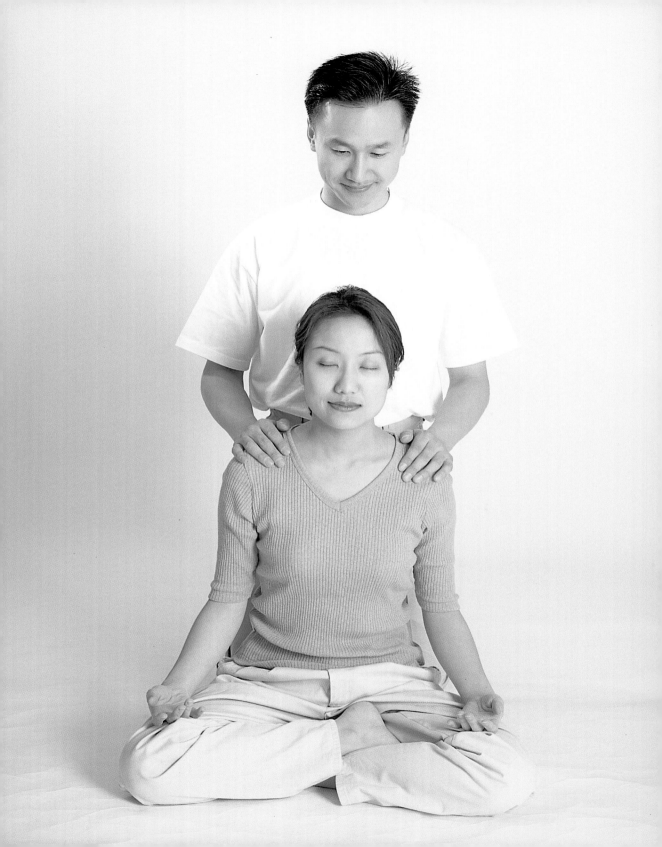

Chapter 12

For Advanced Practitioners

1. Our Bodies: A Miniature Universe
2. Yin Yang, the Five Elements and the Meridians
3. Assessments
4. Bo-Sah-Bup: Strengthening and Dispersing Ki
5. Healing Hands Exercises for Advanced Practitioners

This chapter is for those
who intend to become professional Hwal-
Gong practitioners. However, do not forget
that the most important Hwal-Gong "technique" is a loving mindset.

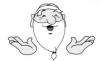

For those who seek expertise in Hwal-Gong, this chapter intro-
duces the basic academic concepts in Oriental Medicine. However,
before going deeply into the theoretic aspects of Hwal-Gong,
remember that most importantly, you must do it with love for your
receiver and for yourself. A practitioner may have exceptional
skills, but if he/she uses it only for personal gain without deference
for the receiver, this cannot be considered Hwal-Gong. Keep in
mind that Hwal-Gong is the act of giving love, and that by utilizing
the following lessons, you will be able to become an excellent Hwal-
Gong practitioner.

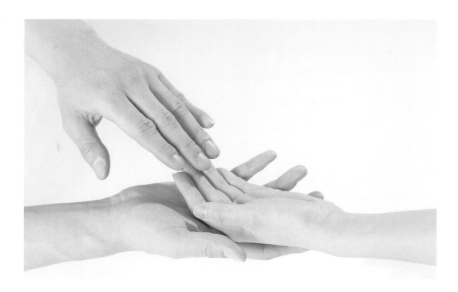

1. Our Bodies: A Miniature Universe

1) Yin Yang, the Five Elements

It is an ancient Asian belief that the harmony between Yin and Yang, as well as the harmonious flow of the Five Elements, created the cosmos. It is also believed that our bodies are miniature replicas of the universe. Of Yin and Yang, the Yin represents characteristics that are feminine, cold, dark, spacious, stagnant, etc. In contrast, Yang represents characteristics that are masculine, hot, bright, time-oriented, pure, etc. One is not better than the other. Rather, their mutual integration and interaction produce balance. For example, there must be night (Yin) in order for day (Yang) to exist; and there must be land (Yin) for sky (Yang) to exist.

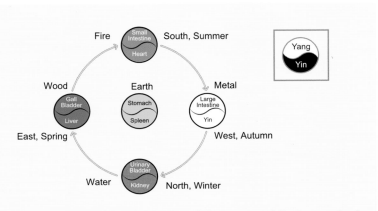

Relationship between the Five elements and the organs of the human body

The Five Elements pertain to Water, Fire, Wood, Metal, and Earth. That which is damp and flows downward is Water. That which burns and heads upward, is Fire. That which is flexible or bendable, yet can remain straight is Wood. A hard, solid and cold object is Metal. Earth is where seeds are sown and benefits are reaped.

2) Five Elements and Organs

The Five Jang (Viscera) inside our bodies are governed by Yin Meridians. Six Bu (Organs) are governed by Yang Meridians. In turn, each of the Five Jang (Viscera) and six Bu (Organs) have Five Elements of their own. Note below the individual functions of viscera and organs.

① Spleen and Stomach

These pertain to Earth. The spleen makes blood and sends Ki and energy from nutrients to the lungs. Problems in the spleen lead to problems in digestion, malnutrition, and similar disorders. The stomach receives food and sends pure nutrients to the spleen; the impure nutrients are sent to the small intestine. Blockage in the Stomach Meridian causes indigestion and diarrhea. After absorbing nutrients, the stomach and spleen, together, make flesh. Those who hesitate before doing anything or are preoccupied with too many thoughts usually have a dysfunction in these meridians.

② Heart and Small Intestine

These are Fire Elements. The heart supplies blood to all of the blood vessels and regulates circulation. The heart also regulates one's mental activity. The lack or excess of fire in the heart can cause anxiety or difficulties in sleeping.

The spleen and small intestine absorb the nutrient energy from the stomach and then send waste to the large intestine to be discharged.

The small intestine is related to the heart. Those who are extremely calm and do not express anger under any circumstances may have a problem in their Heart Meridians.

③ Liver and Gall Bladder

These are Wood Elements. The liver stores blood and softens Ki. It also maintains, protects, and detoxifies our bodies. A dysfunction in the liver can lead to a problem in the muscles. This can also lead to problems in our organs related to the liver, like the reproductive organs, nipples (areola and mammary glands), eyes, ears, and head. Hemorrhaging and irregular menstruation may occur. The gallbladder is related to the Liver Meridian. The gallbladder, as an auxiliary digestive organ, releases bile and assists the liver. A dysfunction in the Gall Bladder will leave a bitter taste in the mouth and cause pain on the side of the trunk and the waist. People who get angry all the time have problems in this meridian. They have difficulty dealing with their anger.

④ Lungs and Large Intestine

These organs are Metal Elements. Lungs breathe in Ki from the air and filter it through the meridians. Lungs help the heart circulate blood and excrete sweat through the skin. Problems in the lungs can cause seemingly unexplainable fatigue and listlessness. This is

Five Elements	Wood	Fire	Earth	Metal	Water	Superficial Fire
Five Jang (Yin)	Liver (Kwol Yin)	Heart (Soh Yin)	Spleen (Tae Yin)	Lungs (Tae Yin)	Kidneys (Soh Yin)	Pericardium (Kwol Yin)
Six Bu (Yang)	Gall Bladder (Soh Yang)	Small Intestine (Tae Yang)	Stomach (Yang Myung)	Large Intestine (Yang Myung)	Urinary Bladder (Tae Yang)	Triple Heater (Soh Yang)
Where it flows	Legs	Arms	Legs	Arms	Legs	Arms

Relationships between Five Jangs, Six Bus and Meridians

because energy is not sent to various parts of the body the way it should. The large intestine eliminates food waste passed on from the small intestine. Problems in the large intestine can lead to constipation, abdominal pain, and diarrhea. People who suffer these problems tend to worry about trivial things. Constant and solitary worrying will cause further damage to this meridian.

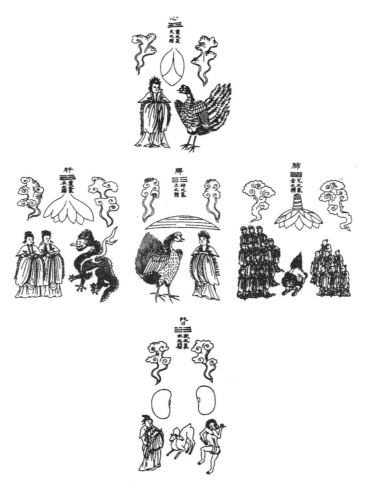

From the medical encyclopedia of Chosun Dynasty of Korea, these figures depict our five major organs. It was believed that each of these organs is protected by its Shin (deity).

⑤ Kidneys and Urinary Bladder

These are Water elements. Since one's birth, the Kidneys store Won-Ki (Inherited strength or energy), and influence physical development and reproductive functions, as well as affects the skeletal system. Kidney problems in children may impede their growth and in adulthood, may lead to sexual dysfunction or hearing problems. The urinary bladder stores unnecessary bodily fluids until eliminating them. Problems in the bladder lead to frequent urination and hematuria. Those who are too frightened to ride on a roller coaster most likely have weak Urinary Bladder Meridians.

⑥ Pericardium Meridian and Triple Heater Meridian

These meridians have names and functions but do not physically exist in our bodies. They are Fire elements, but their greater function is to assist the heart. Therefore, they are considered Superficial Fire. The Pericardium Meridian surrounds the heart (not to be confused with the physical pericardium layers), and governs the heart and lungs. Because the heart and lungs are constantly in motion, the Pericardium Meridian has to prevent friction, and protect against overheating caused by these two ever- active organs. The Triple Heater is not a single meridian. Rather, it is divided into three parts: Upper Heater in the chest, Middle Heater in the upper abdominal, and Lower Heater in the lower abdominal area. The Lower Heater aids the stomach's functions to sustain and protect the body.

3) Five Elements and their Generating and Controlling Cycles

The Five Elements in our bodies maintain checks and balances by reviving and constraining each other. This is known as the Generating and Controlling Cycles.

The Five Elements do not operate by having one particular element's characteristics overwhelm the others. Each of the Five Elements generates some characteristics and at the same time, constrains other characteristics.

① The Generating Cycle – reviving relationships

Wood Generates Fire –Wood allows Fire to burn

Wood enables fire to burn. Looking at our bodies, if the Wood-element organs–liver and gall bladder–efficiently store blood, release clots and detoxify, then the Fire-element organs–heart and small intestine–function properly as well.

Fire Generates Earth–Fire produces soil.

After something is burnt, the remaining ashes become part of the soil. The heart and small intestine (Fire elements) are responsible for distributing Ki and blood to our bodies. When Ki and blood are abundant, the Earth elements–spleen and stomach–function well.

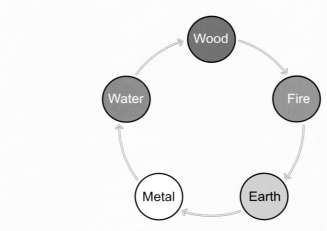

Reviving relationships between the Five Elements

Earth Generates Metal – Metal is found in Earth

From the earth, polished metals can be found. When Earth elements such as the spleen and stomach function well, the digestive system is enhanced. This improves the Metal elements in the lungs and large intestine.

Metal Generates Water – Sweating Rocks

Water's origin is from deep within rocks. Water springs from minerals deep underground. If the Metal-element organs such as the lungs and large intestine function properly, then the Water-element organs, such as the urinary bladder and kidneys' eliminating and reproductive functions will also improve.

Water Generates Wood – Water feeds Trees

Trees draw water from the ground to sustain themselves. The kidneys and bladder, which are Water elements, aid the liver's detoxifying function, and help the Wood-element organs (liver and gall bladder) function better.

② Controlling Cycle - constraining relationships

Wood Controls Earth – Trees use up Earth

Trees sustain themselves by drawing nutrients from the soil. If the Wood-element organs (liver and gall bladder) are overly active, they oppress the energy of the Earth-element organs (spleen and stomach), and thereby weaken the digestive system.

Metal Controls Wood – Metal constrains Wood

Metallic tools such as axes and saws are used to cut wood. Likewise, Metal energy is used to cut up Wood energy. A problem in Metal-element organs would also affect the Wood-element organs. If the lungs do not distribute energy to the body properly, and if the large intestine does not eliminate impure wastes properly, then the liver would have difficulty fulfilling its filtering function.

Water Controls Fire – Water extinguishes Fire

As soon as fire comes in contact with water, it is extinguished. Problems in the Water-element organs – kidneys and bladder – are expressed in the Fire-element organs, the heart and small intestine. Dysfunction in the kidneys or bladder may cause a sudden rise in blood pressure or cause a cardiac arrest.

Fire Controls Metal – Fire molds Metal

Fire has the ability to melt down Metal. Similarly, a problem in Fire-element organs (heart and small intestine) will affect the Metal-element organs (lungs and large intestine) by causing respiratory problems or constipation.

Earth Controls Water – Earth absorbs Water

As the ocean is reclaimed by filling it with soil, the earth soaks up water. Problems in the Earth-element organs (spleen and stomach) can lead to problems in the kidneys and bladder such as dysfunction of the reproductive system or ears.

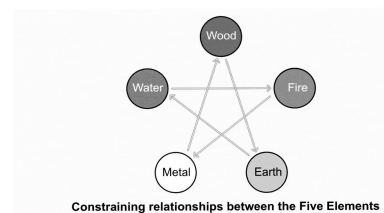

Constraining relationships between the Five Elements

2. Yin Yang, the Five Elements, and the Meridians

1) The Meridians

The meridians, known in Korea as Kyung Rak, are pathways for energy; Kyung refers to vertically flowing meridians, and Rak refers to horizontally flowing meridians. As the meridians intertwine vertically and horizontally, energy is able to reach throughout the body. Kyung Hyul refers to points where Ki enters and exits. They are related to acupressure points.

Kyung Rak flows as follows:

Liver → Lungs → Large Intestine → Stomach → Spleen → Heart → Small Intestine → Urinary Bladder → Kidneys → Triple Heater → Gall Bladder → Liver

In order to be sustained, our bodies must circulate Ki and blood. Ki is Yin and blood is Yang. Ki Hyul flows along Kyung Rak. Ki moves first and the blood follows. If Ki is stagnant, blood does not circulate. In turn, if Ki is ill, blood becomes diseased. If Ki circulates poorly, then blood clots and rots. Ki enters through the breath and blood is produced by food absorption. Poor breathing inhibits proper digestion. Hwal-Gong enhances Ki circulation, and through the meridians, Ki and blood circulations become smooth. A human body has twelve Regular Meridians and eight Extraordinary Meridians. Of the twelve Regular Meridians, six are Yin and the other six are Yang. Of the Yin Meridians, three flow on the arms and the other three flow on the legs. The same applies for Yang

Meridians. When there is an imbalance in the Regular Meridians, the Extraordinary Meridians act as buffers and in general, regulate the system. The fourteen most commonly treated meridians include the twelve Regular Meridians and two Extraordinary Meridians, the Governor and Conception Meridians. This is because the Conception and Governor Meridians are found in the center of our bodies, but the rest of the Extraordinary Meridians are located deep within and their function is to store Ki. Within the fourteen meridians are 365 acupressure points.

The aforementioned meridians - Spleen and Stomach, Heart and Small Intestine, Liver and Gall Bladder, Lungs and Large Intestine, Kidneys and Urinary Bladder, Pericardium and Triple Heater - are connected by the same Kyung Rak. They are divided into Yin and Yang; they balance each other out.

2) Twelve Regular Meridians

The following organs discussed are described in a concept different from Western medicine. They must be understood from a different perspective. For example, Western medicine describes the lungs as oxygen-exchange organs, but in the East, they are perceived in a broader perspective. They are viewed as organs that distribute Ki all throughout the body.

Five Elements	Wood	Fire	Earth	Metal	Water	Supplement Fire
Five Jang (Yin)	Liver (Kwol Yin)	Heart (Soh Yin)	Spleen (Tae Yin)	Lungs (Tae Yin)	Kidneys (Soh Yin)	Pericardium (Kwol Yin)
Six Bu (Yang)	Gall Bladder (Soh Yang)	Small Intestine (Tae Yang)	Stomach (Yang Myung)	Large Intestine (Yang Myung)	Urinary Bladder (Tae Yang)	Triple Heater (Soh Yang)
Where it flows	Legs	Arms	Legs	Arms	Legs	Arms

Relationships between Five Jangs, Six Bus and Meridians

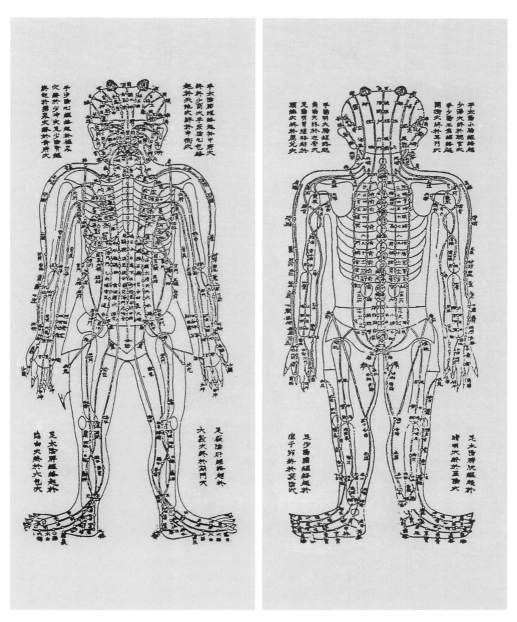

These figures show the flow of the meridian paths. The left figure shows the anterior side, and the right figure shows the posterior side.

① Hand Tae Yin Lung Meridian

The lungs are located above all other internal organs, and they wrap around the other organs like lotus petals. Problems in the lungs can result in flushed faces and dry mouths; they can also cause stuffy chests, neuralgia in arms and wrists, and hot palms. The lungs are responsible for sending Ki to the Five Jang (Viscera) and Six Bu (Organs); therefore, any dysfunction in the lungs will cause a lack of energy and the skin's loss of glow. When such symptoms are present, apply Hwal-Gong along the Lung Meridian. The Lung Meridian runs from the pectoral region down to the tips of the thumbs, and consists of 11 points.

Hand Tae Yin Lung Meridian Path

①This Meridian begins from around the center of the body (internal),

② then runs down through the large intestine.

③ It comes back up, and goes through the diaphragm,

④ and then enters the organs—the lungs.

⑤ After it passes the lungs, it goes up to the neck, pivots down underneath the collarbone, and starts on a myofascial path beginning with the Joong-bu point (Central or Middle Palace).

⑥ Along the fascia and muscles, this meridian runs toward the medial section of the arm.

⑦ It passes the elbow and over the radial nerves on the wrists,

⑧ and continues on to the hands to the tips of the thumbs.

⑨ A branch of the Lung Meridian splits from immediately above the wrists, and runs to the index finger, where the Large Intestine Meridian begins.

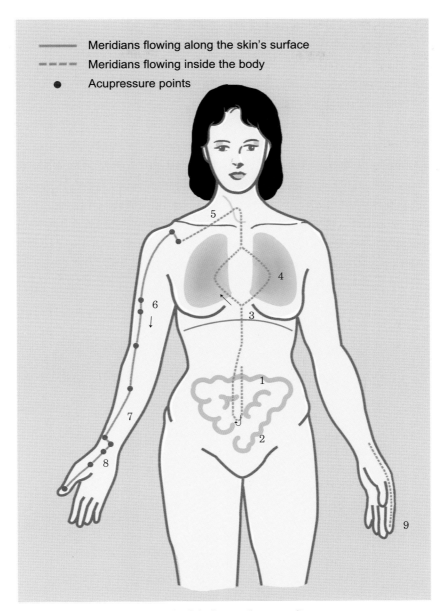

Meridians flowing along the skin's surface
Meridians flowing inside the body
● Acupressure points

• The numbers correspond to the labeling on the opposite page.
• Although the diagram shows the meridian only on one side of the body, the Twelve Meridians exist bilaterally.

② **Hand Yang Myung Large Intestine Meridian**

The large intestine starts with the Su-boon point (1 inch above the navel). It overlaps with the small intestine sixteen times, and then connects with the anus. The large intestine removes wastes. Their dysfunction will cause toothaches, stuffy noses, frequent nosebleeds and sore throats. Stuffy chests and hand and wrist neuralgia may occur, as well. The Large Intestine Meridian begins at the cuticles of the index fingers, and runs along the radial side toward the elbows, and then passes through the shoulder blades. From there, it passes the neck bones and a depression on the collarbone, to deep down into the lungs. After passing the lungs, this meridian goes down to the large intestine. The meridian that branched from the clavicle passes the cheeks, goes around the mouth, and ends between the nose and the mouth.

Hand Yang Myung Large Intestine Meridian Path

① The Large Intestine Meridian starts on the dorsum of the hands and on the radial sides of the index fingers.

② It passes between the first and second metacarpals, then to the wrists, and goes up along the arms.

③ After it passes the elbows (now closer to the torso), this meridian flows near the ulnar sides of the arms

④ up to the point where the shoulders meet the neck,

⑤ and then splits into two branches.

⑥ One of these branches goes deep inside the body and through the lungs,

⑦ then passes through the diaphragm, and enters the large intestine.

⑧ The other branch climbs up the neck along the myofascial surface,

⑨ then passes the cheeks.

⑩ One branch goes deep into the gums, and the myofascial line goes around the upper lip, and ends on the side of nostril (on the opposite side).

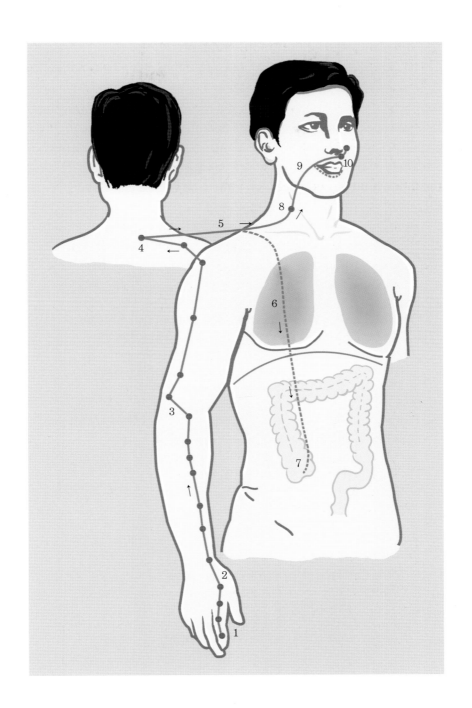

③ Foot Yang Myung Stomach Meridian

The stomach, located on the upper abdomen, is an essential organ that controls digestion. Problems in the stomach can cause headaches, especially around the forehead, and in the supraorbital and the occipital regions. Other symptoms include rash or hives around the mouth, abdominal pains, paraesthesia, or stiffness in the knees and legs. In more severe cases, symptoms include dry lips, loss of appetite, acid dyspepsia, gastric ulcer, and gastritis.

Foot Yang Myung Stomach Meridian Path

① The Stomach Meridian starts from where the Large Intestine Meridian ends.
② It follows along the sides of the nose up to the medial corners of the eyes, and then meets up with the Urinary Bladder Meridian. It goes back down along the sides of the nose to the upper gums.
③ It returns to the lips and to the chin, follows along the jaws,
④ then goes up past the front of the ears, and ends there.
⑤ A meridian branching off from the chin
⑥ goes down toward the torso and deep into the stomach, then it connects to the spleen.
⑦ Another branch follows along the facial sheath,
⑧ passes the abdomen, and goes to the pubis.
⑨ Inside the body, below the stomach, it begins another internal meridian branch; goes down the abdomen,
⑩ and meets with the myofascial meridian from the pubis.
⑪ The merged meridians run down the front of the thighs
⑫ to the lateral sides of the knees.
⑬ Then, it follows along the outside (fibula side) of the legs, and ends on the second toes.
⑭ Below the knees, another set of lines branch off and end on the third toes. Another set of lines branch off from the dorsum of feet, and connect with the big toes and the Spleen Meridian.

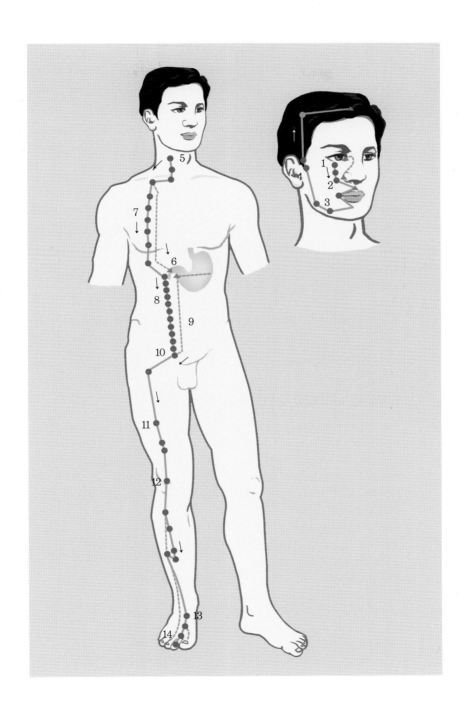

④ Foot Tae Yin Spleen Meridian

This is a digestive meridian focusing mainly on the spleen but also includes the pancreas. This meridian also has an intimate relationship with the ovaries and uterus. In the East, it is believed that the spleen heats up the Five Jang (Viscera) and the stomach, thereby aiding digestion. The spleen is Yin and the stomach is Yang; together they create the Yin Yang balance.

Problems in the Spleen Meridian cause stiffness in the tongue, heaviness in the upper stomach area accompanied by severe pain, nausea and frequent diarrhea or constipation. The legs may also feel very heavy. Menstrual irregularity or abnormal hemorrhaging in the uterus may occur in females.

Foot Tae Yin Spleen Meridian Path

① The Spleen Meridian begins on the tibia sides of the big toes, and goes along the medial borders of the feet;

② it passes the front of the medial malleolus, and goes up along the medial borders of the legs.

③ It continues to follow the medial aspect of the knees and thighs toward the top of the body.

④ It enters the abdomen,

⑤ The internal meridian passes through the spleen,

⑥ and connects to the stomach.

⑦ The myofascial meridian continues upward and ends on the chest.

⑧ Then the meridian goes up the neck,

⑨ and ends at the base of the tongue to disperse Ki and blood.

⑩ The meridian that leaves the stomach continues onto the heart and begins the Heart Meridian.

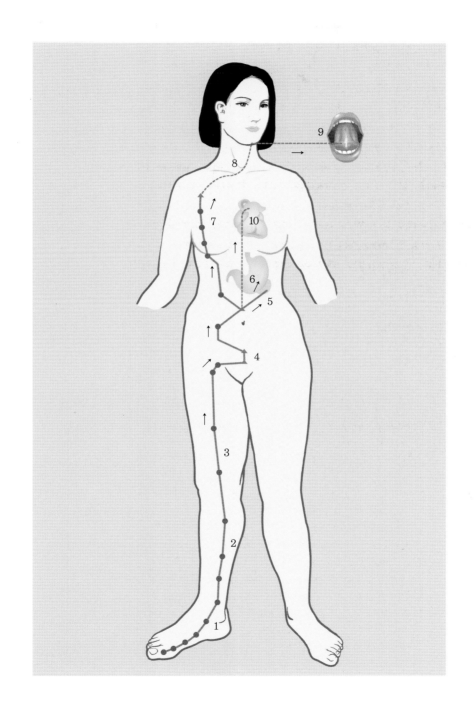

⑤ Hand Soh Yin Heart Meridian

The heart is an organ shaped like a lotus bulb. It is located below the lungs close to the fifth thoracic vertebra. Problems in the heart can lead to frequent thirst and red eyes. There may be pain or neuralgia in the little fingers, as well. The palms may feel painful. The face may become flushed, and the sufferer may experience insomnia. People with heart problems smile easily, and tend to be anxious.

The Heart Meridian begins at the heart, goes around the small intestine with one line branching out from the axilla (under arm), and ends in the little fingers.

Hand Soh Yin Heart Meridian Path

① The Heart Meridian is a group of three branches of meridians that begin from the heart.
② One of these branches flows past the diaphragm, and connects to the small intestine.
③ Another branch goes up and connects to the eyes.
④ The remaining branch passes through the lungs,
⑤ penetrates the axilla, and flows along the ulnar sides of the arms,
⑥ continues on along the ulna,
⑦ passes the wrists and palms, and ends in the tips of the little fingers.

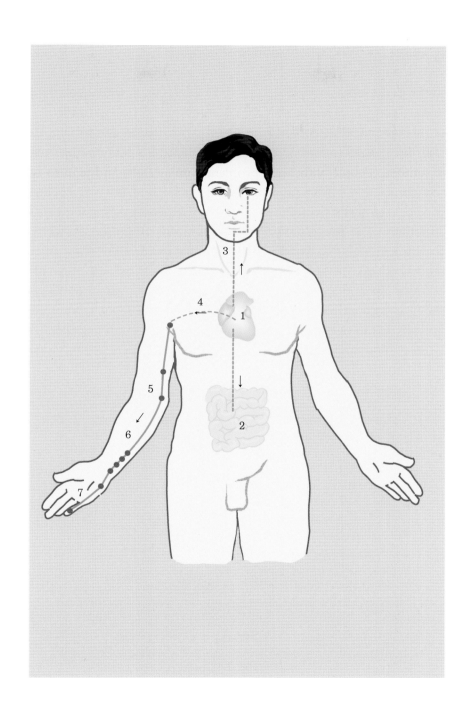

⑥ Hand Tae Yang Small Intestine Meridian

The small intestine, located below the stomach and encircled by the large intestine, is 13 to 20 feet in length. This is where pure and impure properties are separated; the liquid waste is sent to the urinary bladder, and the solids are sent to the large intestine. An unhealthy small intestine can result in yellowish sclera and hearing impairment. Additional symptoms include swelling of the cheeks, sore throat and stiffness in the back of the neck. Men may experience pain in their testes, and women may experience irregular menstruations. The Small Intestine Meridian begins on the dorsal side of the little fingers, continues to the elbows toward the shoulders, zigzags across the scapulas, and goes past the shoulders to Gyulboon (a dip in the collarbone). One branch travels down through the heart; the other goes up to the face toward the ears. A third branch goes to the medial corners of the eyes, and connects with the Urinary Bladder Meridian.

Hand Tae Yang Small Intestine Meridian Path

① The Small Intestine Meridian begins on the dorsal side of the hands–the ulnar sides of the little fingers.
② This meridian continues up toward the ulnar sides of the forearms
③ and the upper arms (toward the little fingers),
④ travels up to the top center of the back (where it meets up with the Governor Meridian),
⑤ lands on the clavicle, and splits into two branches.
⑥ The branch going into the chest connects with the heart,
⑦ passes through the diaphragm,
⑧ and goes into the small intestine.
⑨ The other branch travels on the front and side of the neck along with the carotid artery toward the face,
⑩ passes the cheeks,
⑪ touches the lateral corners of the eyes, and goes to the ears.
⑫ Another branch from the cheeks goes to the medial corners of the eyes, and connects with the Urinary Bladder Meridian.

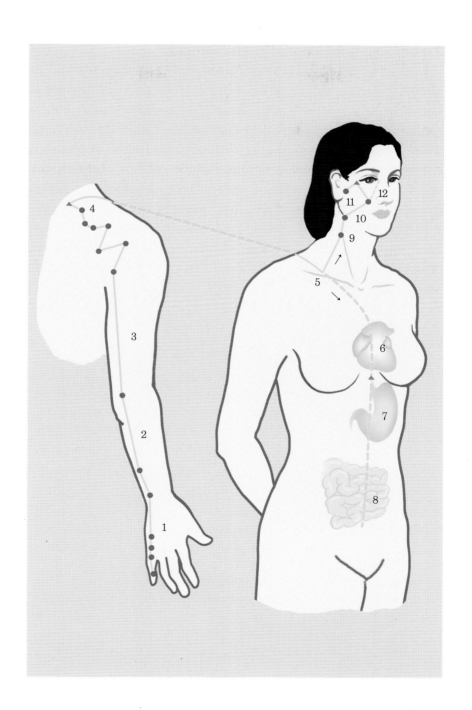

⑦ Foot Tae Yang Urinary Bladder Meridian

Of the 14 meridians discussed in this chapter, the Urinary Bladder Meridian is the longest, and has the most number of points. Therefore, this meridian contains many essential points. This is the Eastern perspective on the urinary bladder: After food is digested in the stomach, nutrients are absorbed in the small intestine, and the remaining fluid is accumulated in the urinary bladder. Problems in the Urinary Bladder Meridian cause somewhat unique symptoms. Aside from headaches caused by overworking, they may cause nosebleeds and pain in the waist, arms, legs, and shoulders. In severe cases, the legs may become paralyzed. In addition, there may be problems in the respiratory, circulatory, digestive, or reproductive systems.

Foot Tae Yang Urinary Bladder Meridian Path

① This meridian begins at the medial corners of the eyes and travels up the forehead toward the top of the head.
② From there, a small line branches off and enters the brain.
③ The main line continues to travel down the back of the head.
④ At the back of the neck, this line spits in two.
⑤ The medial branch goes down to the seventh cervical vertebra,
⑥ and follows straight down the spine, but
⑦ at the lumbar area, an internal line goes in to connect with the kidneys.
⑧ It then goes into the urinary bladder.
⑨ The other line (from the neck) comes down the back of the shoulders,
⑩ travels down very close to the medial branch of the Urinary Bladder Meridian and to the gluteal region.
⑪ These two braches travel down the posterior thighs,
⑫ merge at the popliteal regions, and continue down on the posterior sides of the legs.
⑬ The merged line goes around the lateral malleolus, and ends in the little toes.

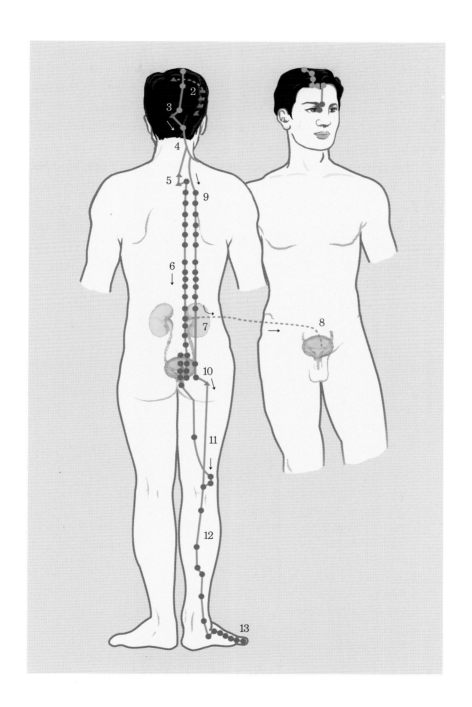

⑧ Foot Soh Yin Kidney Meridian

According to Eastern medicine, the kidneys include the adrenal structures believed to contain Won-Ki and Jung, the innate life energy. It is said that about half of a person's weight is water, and the crucial organs that produce this water are the kidneys and the adrenals.

The first symptom of a weak Kidney Meridian is discomfort in the waist. The face loses luster and color, the mouth does not produce a sufficient amount of saliva, and one experiences shortness of breath. The sufferers feel hunger without having an appetite; their health deteriorates, and they have frequent diarrhea.

The Kidney Meridian begins in the middle of the feet (plantar surface), travels up the medial sides of the legs, and passes the kidneys to end just below the neck.

Foot Soh Yin Kidney Meridian Path

① This Meridian begins from beneath the little toes, travels across the soles of the feet,

② circles around the medial malleolus,

③ and travels up the medial sides of the legs.

④ It continues to travel up the medial sides of the thighs.

⑤ Near the tail bone, it enters the inner part of the body

⑥ toward the kidneys,

⑦ connects to the urinary bladder,

⑧ and returns to the myofascial surface around the pubis, and then goes up the abdomen toward the chest.

⑨ Another branch exits from the kidneys

⑩ goes past the liver,

⑪ enters the lungs,

⑫ and ends in the tongue.

⑬ Yet another branch from the lungs crosses the heart, and connects to the Pericardium Meridian.

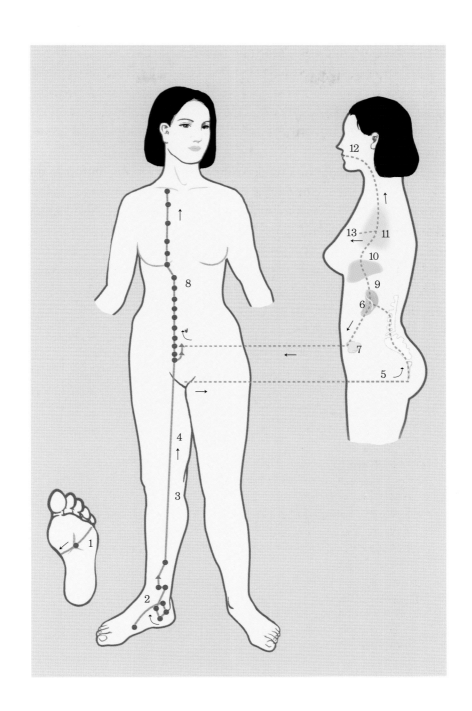

⑨Hand Kwol Yin Pericardium Meridian

The pericardium surrounds the heart like a sac and protects it from negative external energies. The Pericardium Meridian does not represent a physiological organ. This meridian interweaves through out the body, protects the heart and exists as a nonphysical entity that governs the heart.

There are many similarities between problems in the Pericardium Meridian and problems in the Heart Meridian. Problems in the Pericardium Meridian cause a flushed face, palpitation, yellowing of sclera, and spasms in the chest and waist. There may also be pain in the palms or medial sides of the arms. The Pericardium Meridian begins in the chest, and splits into three regions; the chest, upper abdomen, and lower abdomen. One of those branches goes to the side of the chest and runs along the inner side of the arms to terminate in the middle fingers.

Hand Kwol Yin Pericardium Meridian Path

① This meridian begins from the middle of the chest, goes through the pericardium,

② and connects with the Triple Heater Meridian via the diaphragm.

③ Another branch goes across the chest and exits the body through the ribcage.

④ Afterward, it goes around the axilla to the deltoid muscles, and from there

⑤ runs down along the midline of the anterior of the arms (on the Yin or palmar surface).

⑥ On the forearms, this line runs between the Lung and Heart Meridians,

⑦ toward the palms,

⑧ and ends in the tips of the middle fingers. Another branch from the middle of the palms heads to the ring fingers to connect with the Triple Heater Meridian.

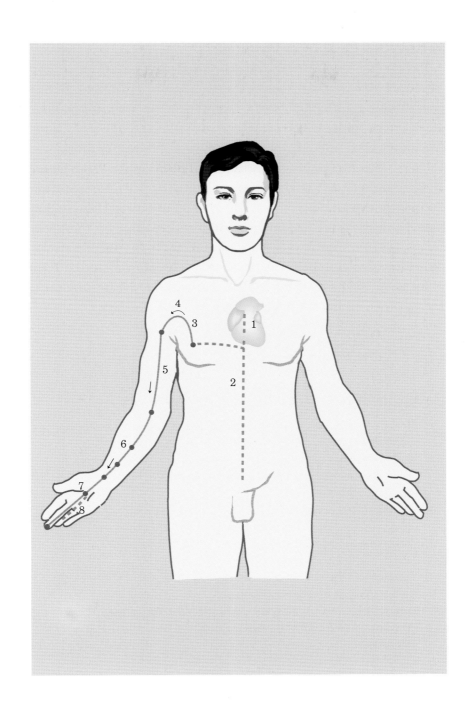

⑩ Hand Soh Yang Triple Heater

The Triple Heater Meridian is paired with the Pericardium Meridian. Like its partner, Pericardium Meridian, the Triple Heater does not have a physical form. From below the neck to the solar plexus is the Upper Heater; from the solar plexus to the navel is the Middle Heater; and the lower abdomen is known as the Lower Heater. These three Heaters form the Triple Heater. The Upper Heater regulates the circulatory system; the Middle Heater regulates the respiratory and digestive systems; and the Lower Heater regulates the reproductive and discharge systems. Problems in the Upper Heater leads to shortness of breath; problems in the Middle Heater causes gas (due to dysfunction of the stomach and liver) and stiffness in the lower abdomen; and problems in the Lower Heater can cause reproductive dysfunctions.

Hand Soh Yang Triple Heater Path

① This meridian begins at the tips of the ring fingers, and follows the dorsum of the hands.

② It continues up the forearms,

③ and goes around the elbows and the upper arms.

④ From the shoulders,

⑤ it travels to the anterior shoulders,

⑥ and goes deep into the chest into the Pericardium

⑦ past the diaphragm, and connects with the Triple Heater.

⑧ This branch exits the body again to run up to the neck,

⑨ goes behind the ears,

⑩ enters the face, and goes deep down.

⑪ From behind the ears, a small line branches out. Via the ears, it goes to the lateral corners of the eyes to connect with the Gall Bladder Meridian.

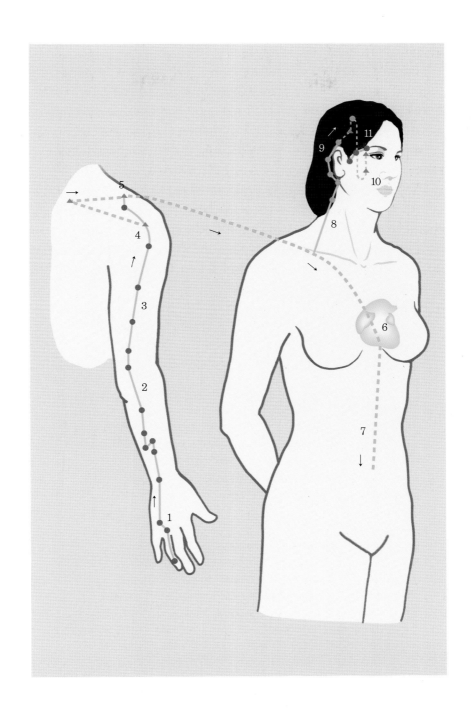

⑪ Foot Soh Yang Gall Bladder Meridian

The Gall Bladder aids liver functions. It is located near the tenth thoracic vertebra and takes up a large area. If problems occur in the liver or gall bladder, the sclera of the eyes turns bluish purple causing general weakness in the eyes accompanied by weakening in the voice. Additional symptoms include dizziness, headaches and fatigue.

The Gall Bladder Meridian runs from head to toe. It begins at the corners of the eyes to the sides of the head. One branch goes to the shoulders and the other one goes into the ears. This branch meets up with the branch that goes around the liver. The original branch goes to the sides of the torso and down the legs, ending in the fourth toe on each foot.

🐢 Foot Soh Yang Gall Bladder Meridian Path ━━━━━

① This meridian begins at the lateral corners of the eyes, and splits into two branches.

② One branch runs back and forth from the face to the temporal regions of the head to behind the ears and down toward the back.

③ It then passes the shoulders, and goes to the axilla,

④ runs along the lateral thorax to the hips.

⑤ Another branch goes into the cheeks

⑥ down the neck

⑦ and the chest,

⑧ connects with the liver, and goes into the gall bladder.

⑨ This line continues down to the lower abdominal region, exits on the myofascial surface, and meets up with the other branch.

⑩ This merged line continues down the lateral sides of the legs,

⑪ passes in front of the lateral malleolus,

⑫ and ends in the fourth toes. From below the lateral malleolus, a small line branches off to the big toes to connect with the Liver Meridian.

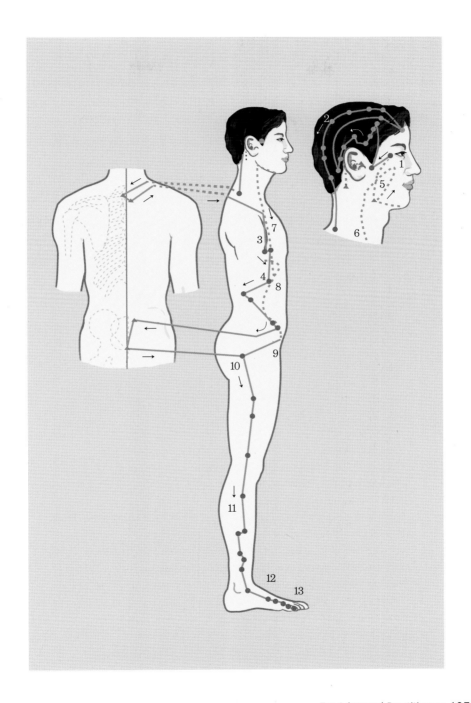

⑫ Foot Kwol Yin Liver Meridian

The liver is located around the ninth thoracic vertebra. This meridian circles around the liver, which detoxifies and maintains the muscles and the joints. People with healthy Liver Meridians are confident and fearless.

Weakness in Liver Meridian causes loss of glow in the face, dry mouths, nausea, and feelings of stuffiness. The big toes may also feel painful. Women may experience cricks in their backs and experience reproductive dysfunctions.

The Liver Meridian begins underneath the big toenails, and goes up across the Kidney and Spleen Meridians. It continues to the pelvic region, crosses the reproductive organs, and goes around and above the gall bladder.

Foot Kwol Yin Liver Meridian Path

① The Liver Meridian begins underneath the big toenail.
② It passes in front of the medial malleolus,
③ runs up the medial sides of the lower extremities,
④ passes the external genitalia,
⑤ heads to the abdominal region, and enters the inner parts of the body.
⑥ It then connects with the liver,
⑦ goes to the gall bladder, and goes sideways along the trunk.
⑧ It enters the lungs (where the meridian cycle starts again),
⑨ goes up the neck,
⑩ lingers at the eyes, and splits into two lines.
⑪ One branch goes down, the other circles around the mouth,
⑫ and the other one goes up to the very top of the head.

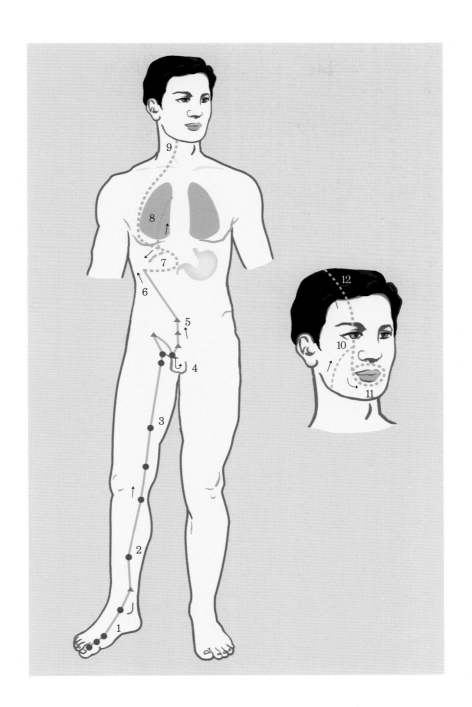

⑬ The Governor Meridian

Of all Extraordinary Meridians, only the Governor Meridian and Conception Meridian are included with the 12 Regular Meridians to comprise the commonly known 14 meridians.

The Governor Meridian and Conception Meridian flow vertically on the anterior and posterior central surfaces of the body. The Governor Meridian promotes good energy circulation. Located along the back, it regulates and oversees the Yang Meridians.

Problems in the Governor Meridian can cause headaches, indigestion, respiratory diseases, or dysfunction of the reproductive system.

The Governor Meridian is a pathway through which the Water energy of the kidneys rise. Therefore, a healthy Governor Meridian will help to cool and clear the head. Water energy goes down to the heart and sends heat from the heart to Dahn-jon. This is the Su-Seung-Hwa-Gang cycle.

The Governor Meridian Path

① The Governor Meridian begins in the pelvic cavity,
② In Females, it goes around and down to the urethra around the tailbone.
③ In males, the Yin Meridian goes down and up on the center of the sacrum.
④ This line continues up the center of the spine.
⑤ It passes the neck and continues to the center of the face.
⑥ It then passes in between the eyes, runs down the center of the bridge of the nose, and ends on In-joong.

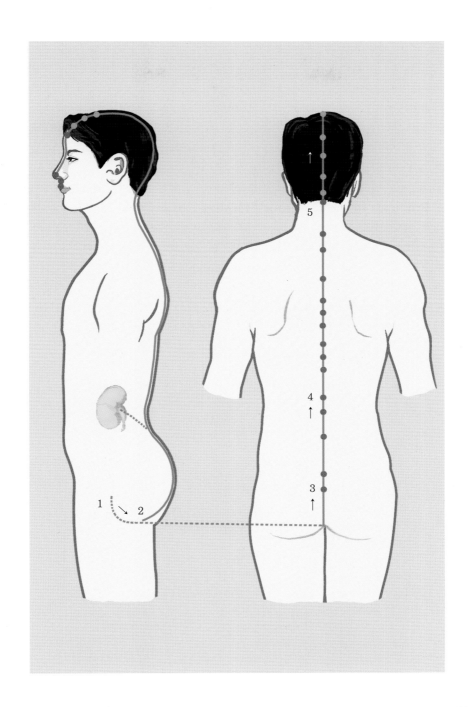

⑭ The Conception Meridian

The Conception Meridian supervises and oversees the Yin Meridians located on the anterior surface of the body. The Conception Meridian passes through the neck and the chest and connects to the lower abdomen. Problems in the Conception Meridian can cause various symptoms, specifically related to pregnancy and labor.

A dysfunctional Conception Meridian causes stiffness in the lower abdomen, menstrual irregularities, and infertility. The heat from the heart travels down to Dahn-jon through the Conception Meridian. Energy blockages in the Conception Meridian can cause heat to rise to the head and consequently cause various illnesses.

The Conception Meridian Path

① This meridian starts at the very center and tip of the pelvic cavity.
② It goes down to the perineum around the pubes,
③ passes the navel,
④ and runs up the center of the chest.
⑤ It goes up the neck to the chin,
⑥ circles around the mouth, and meets up with the Governor Meridian at In-joong point.
⑦ It then passes both the nostrils and meets up with the Stomach Meridian by entering the eyes.

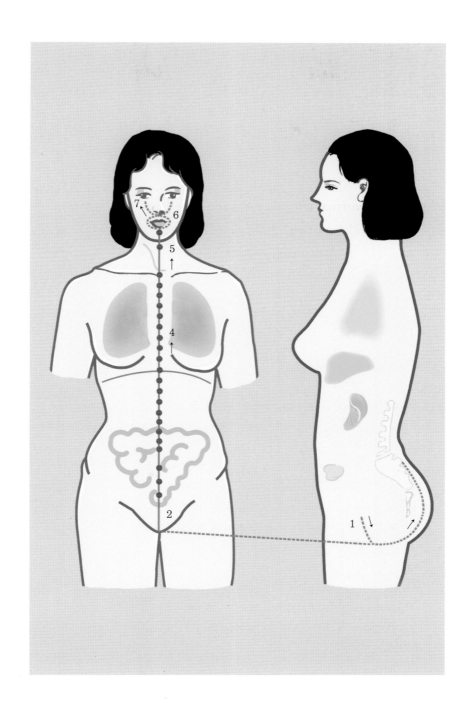

3. Assessments

Finding out the origin and cause of an illness enhances the results of Hwal-Gong. While observing the receiver, it is important to note the receiver's daily habits, such as the amount of walking and his/her postures. However, since hasty judgments may actually cause harm, be sure to include visual, tactile, auditory, and olfactory assessments while taking the receiver's medical history into account. Consider all of the factors seriously to make a holistic assessment.

1) A Visual Assessment

① Check for anterior-posterior and left-right alignments.
- In kneeling: if the right leg is shorter, there is a tendency for constipation.
- Longer left leg may indicate digestive problems.
- Longer right leg may indicate circulatory and respiratory problems.
- Significant variation in thickness in the thoracic region may cause insomnia. Those with thinner left thorax may suffer from nightmares.
- Waist bent forward may indicate digestive problems.
- Depressed chest may indicate heart problems.
- Elevated shoulders may indicate respiratory problems and illness in the lungs.

② Observe coloring

- Pale coloring: those with pale skin and a weak disposition are susceptible to respiratory and digestive dysfunction. Their throats swell easily; they suffer from asthma and constantly feel stuffiness in their chests. These people also have weak stomachs, and therefore, suffer from frequent diarrhea. Their cold hands and feet are accompanied by neuralgia.
- Red coloring: redness in the face and other parts of the body indicates circulation problems. These people experience heart palpitations, shortness of breath, difficulty in walking up and down stairs, and weak small intestinal function.
- Yellow coloring: this may indicate problems in the digestive system accompanied by loss of appetite and eczema.
- Green coloring: people with green skin tones have weak livers, tend to erupt in anger, and often lack courage. They fear much and tire easily.
- Dark coloring: lack of luster and unclean facial complexion indicate problems in the Kidney Meridian. There may be problems in the urinary bladder, as well.

2) Listening and Smelling

- One's voice volume depends on his/her lungs. A faint voice is indicative of weak Ki.
- Psychological discomfort, such as anxiety and nervousness, due to a weak heart can manifest in nonsensical rambling.
- A subtle squeaky sound indicates a possible problem in the gall bladder.
- A body odor may be indicative of diabetes or a hot temper.

3) Ask and Listen

Ask where and when pain is experienced and compare the receiver's past and current symptoms. In addition, compare the conditions before and after each Hwal-Gong session. It is also important to ask about the receiver's occupation, diet, daily activities, and habits. For elderly receivers, tactfully ask about their urinary patterns and digestive conditions. For children, ask if they dream often and whether they have nightmares.

4) Touch

With your receiver standing, touch his/her spine to check his/her alignment and observe the lengths of the legs. With your receiver seated, carefully observe the shoulders to check their alignment. Since the abdomen is a sensitive region, be careful not to press it abruptly or hard. First, start with your hands relaxed, and then gradually increase the pressure. Those who have stiffness around their navels have problems in their stomachs, spleens, and have hardened large intestine. For these receivers, apply Hwal-Gong on their legs along the Spleen Meridians. Stiffness below the navel indicates a problem in the kidneys. The solar plexus, the area above the navel, is related to the arm's Pericardium Meridian. Thus, stiffness in this region indicates a problem in the heart.

4. Strengthening and Dispersing Ki: Bo-Sah-Bup

Bo Sah Bup is a technique used to discern whether a problem area has an excessive or deficient amount of energy flow. Appropriately treat the area by increasing or decreasing the energy levels. Imbalance in Ki is not healthy; neither too much or too little Ki is good.

1) Bo Bup for Symptoms of Weakness

When someone is malnourished, he/she appears weak. Symptoms of weakness refer to the lack in Ki. Receivers with symptoms showing weakness have weak Ki or dispersed Ki. Thus, it is important to replenish them with a sufficient amount of Ki. When treating weak areas, do not apply Sah Bup or intense pressures. Intense pressure on a weak person or on sensitive areas like the abdomen is like taking away the last drop of energy from a person who hardly has any.

Apply Bo Bup by pressing with palms or gentle smoothing. With this technique, pressure is not concentrated on a small area. Even when you use your thumbs, do not press hard. When treating receivers with weakness symptoms, it may be enough for you to simply lay your hands on him/her.

2) Sah Bup for Symptoms Showing Excess Ki

Symptoms showing an excess amount of Ki manifest when too much Ki in an area constricts a natural flow of energy. This type of blockage can prevent negative energy from leaving the body. In this situation, Bo Bup or increased energy will not alleviate the symptoms. In the areas of excess, use your thumbs or elbows to apply "almost painful" amounts of pressure. In doing so, you are releasing negative energy and releasing the blockages.

3) Applying Bo Sah for Hwal-Gong

A person may have weak or excessive energy, however the entire bodily system including the Five Jang (Viscera) Six Bu (Organs) cannot automatically be assumed to have the corresponding conditions. If one part of our body is low in energy, then another part of our body will have excessive amounts of energy. For example, if the kidneys - Water elements - are too weak, then the organs that generate the Metal elements may be over stimulated, and the energy of the Water element will be further depleted. So, apply Sah Bup (calming) to the lungs and the large intestine–the Metal elements– and apply Bo Bup (strengthening) to the heart and small intestine –the Fire elements (which have a controlling relationship with Water).

This is merely the basics of an intricate theory. Understanding the weak/excessive conditions of Jang (Viscera) and Bu (Organs) requires a great amount of experience and study. This is not to say that becoming a Hwal-Gong practitioner requires you to study Oriental medicine. However, if you know the basic theory and principles, you will not have any trouble applying Hwal-Gong in your daily life.

Below are some techniques for Hwal-Gong.

① If lightly pressing an area causes pain, that area has excessive energy, nervousness, and blocked energy. If energy is excessively concentrated in one point that means negative energy is intent on remaining in the body. It is fighting not to leave. In this case, simply releasing the meridian points will help your body to recover quickly.

② On the contrary, if a person shows no significant reactions to hard pressures other than feeling good, that person's body is weak. At the same time, the body's defense system has become weak. In this case, it is important to supplement his/her energy level.

③ In order to restore normal sensitivities to such receivers, it is important to have applied Hwal-Gong on many people. It is important to build academic knowledge about Hwal-Gong. However, it is more important to develop sensitivity in your hands. Once you become an expert, you will not only be able to calm excess energy, but also strengthen the corresponding weak areas by pressing one's painful areas.

④ As mentioned earlier, in Hwal-Gong, you should not press on another's body absentmindedly. Pay special attention to receivers with chronic or serious medical conditions. Follow the Bo Sah Bup principles.

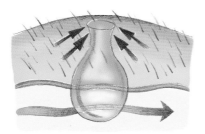

Clogged Hyul
- symptoms of excess.
This is a state when excessive energy is accumulated in one point. Use thumbs or elbows to stimulate; or tap with your fists.

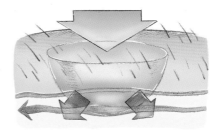

Wide open Hyul
- symptoms of weakness.
This is a state when energy is weak and dispersed. Press or smooth with palms to increase energy.

5. Healing Hands Exercises for Advanced Practitioners

In order to turn your hands into healing hands, your body must be in its best health condition, so that the body itself can supply its own medicine. Avoid overworking and overeating. Do Dahn-jon breathing and healing hands exercises diligently for 21 days. A good physical condition indicates that your state of mind is always joyous and peaceful. The best way to turn your hands into healing hands is by opening your heart and mind the best you can and by having a loving heart. Note the following exercises.

1 Fully relax your body, and sit in a half or full lotus position.

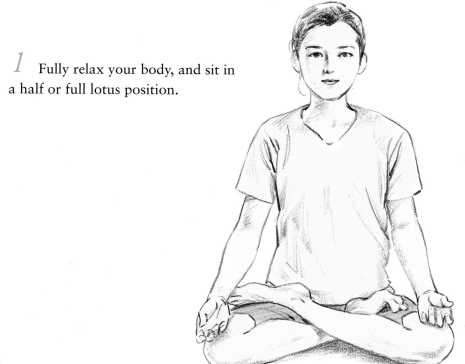

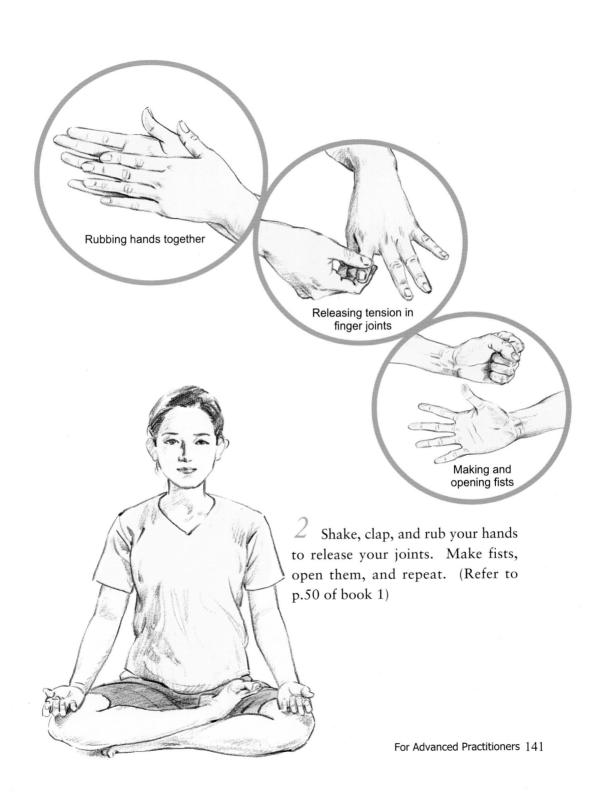

Rubbing hands together

Releasing tension in
finger joints

Making and
opening fists

2 Shake, clap, and rub your hands
to release your joints. Make fists,
open them, and repeat. (Refer to
p.50 of book 1)

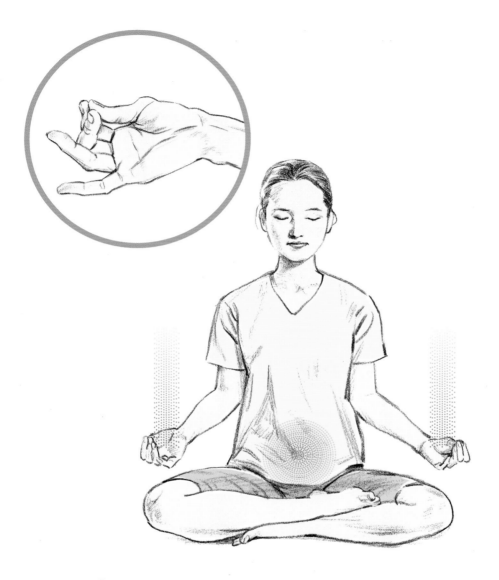

3 Bring the first three fingers of each hand together to a point.
Place your hands about 4 inches above the knees.

4 Focus on Dahn-jon. Picture strong beams of energy entering
your palms.

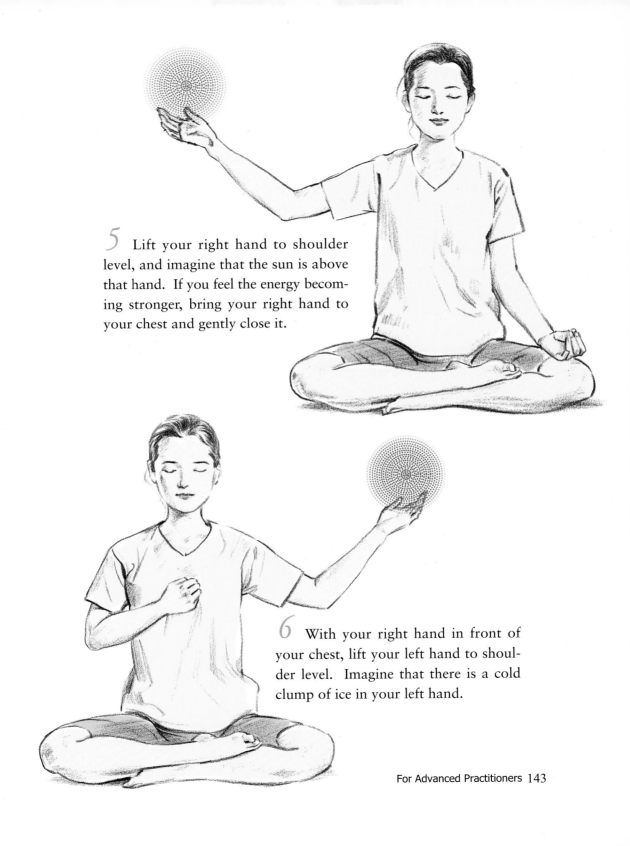

5 Lift your right hand to shoulder level, and imagine that the sun is above that hand. If you feel the energy becoming stronger, bring your right hand to your chest and gently close it.

6 With your right hand in front of your chest, lift your left hand to shoulder level. Imagine that there is a cold clump of ice in your left hand.

7 When you are able to feel the sensations growing, bring your palms together as though in prayer up to your eyebrows. Begin meditating in this posture. Through both your hands, feel the sensations throughout your body. You may feel that your chest is dividing into two (left and right) and other parts of your body are separating as well. Remain in this position for 40 minutes. When starting, It may be too difficult to maintain this posture for 40 minutes, so start with 5 minutes in the beginning, and then gradually increase to 40 minutes.

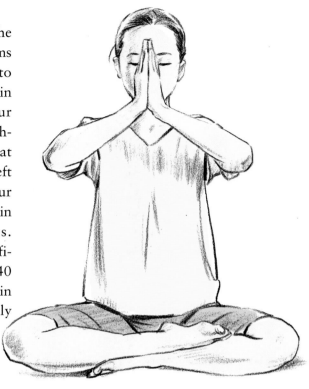

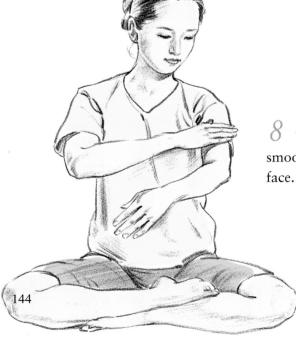

8 To finish, clap 30 times, and smooth down your chest, arms and face.

144

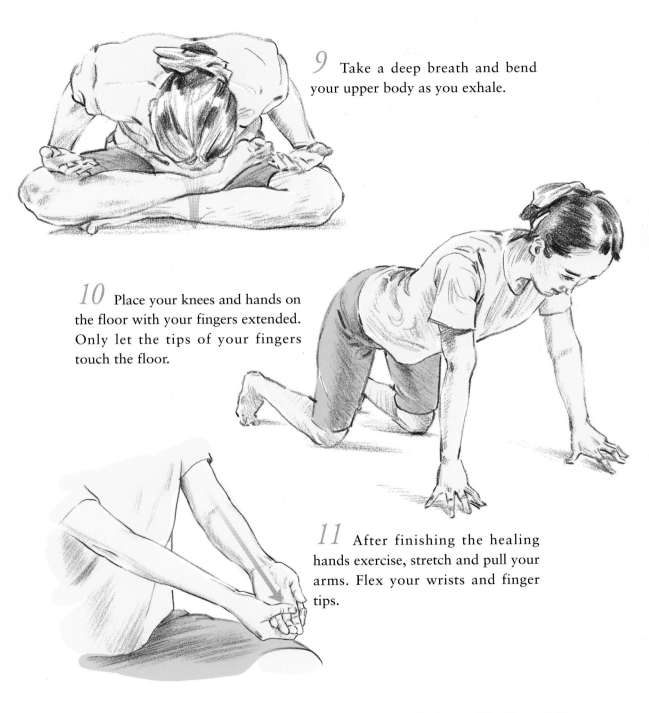

9 Take a deep breath and bend your upper body as you exhale.

10 Place your knees and hands on the floor with your fingers extended. Only let the tips of your fingers touch the floor.

11 After finishing the healing hands exercise, stretch and pull your arms. Flex your wrists and finger tips.

Abdominal cramps_30, 40, 43

Anxiety_26, 40, 43

Arthritis_52, 61

Bloating_52

Bronchitis_26, 83

Chest pain_15, 26

Colon dysfunction_83

Constipation_30, 33, 37, 40, 83

Coughing_33

Depression_26, 33, 37

Diabetes_37, 43

Diarrhea_30, 33, 56

Dysentery_30

Dysmenorrhea_37, 43

Eczema_56

Fatigue_17, 33, 37, 40, 52, 59, 66, 74, 77

Frozen shoulders_15, 83

Gastric ptosis_43

Gastric ulcer_33, 37, 43

Gastritis_43, 59

Headache_26, 52, 74

Heart disease_77

Hemiplegia_80

Hepatitis_56

Hypertension_43, 66

Indigestion_26, 37, 40, 74, 83

Inflammation of papillae (or tongue)_33

Inflammation of reproductive organs_52

Insomnia_33, 37

Knees arthritis_80

Leg pain_56

Loss of appetite_33

Menstrual cramps_30

Menstrual irregularity_33

Nervousness_26, 40

Neuralgia_80

Pain and sprain in the knees_61

Pain in arms_77

Paralysis in lower extremities_80

Peptic disorders_26

Peptic ulcer_59

Pneumonia_83

Raynaud's syndrome_33

Shoulder pain_15, 74, 77, 83

Stomach dysfunction_83

Symptoms of cholecystitis_56

Uteritis_30

Vomiting_33, 43